Practical Quantitative Doppler Echocardiography

Author
John H. Phillips

With the Assistance of
Willie Sessions, M.D.
Senior Cardiology Research Fellow

CRC Press
Boca Raton Ann Arbor Boston London

Library of Congress Cataloging-in-Publication Data

Phillips, John H.
Practical quantitative Doppler echocardiography / John H. Phillips; with the assistance of Willie Sessions.
p. cm.
Includes bibliographical references and index.
ISBN 0-8493-4921-4
1. Doppler echocardiography. I. Sessions, Willie. II. Title.
[DNLM: 1. Echocardiography, Doppler. WG 141.5.E2 P561p]
RC 683.5.U5P49 1991
616.1′207′543—dc20
DNLM/DLC
for Library of Congress
91-23358

CIP

Direct all inquiries to CRC Press, Inc., 2000 Corporate Blvd., N. W., Boca Raton, Florida, 33431.

International Standard Book Number 0-8493-4921-4

Library of Congress Card Number 91-23358
Printed in the United States 4 5 6 7 8 9 0
Printed on acid-free paper

PREFACE

Doppler echocardiography has become extremely valuable in the diagnosis and management of a large number of patients with cardiovascular diseases. This technology is now an essential part of any modern, noninvasive cardiology laboratory. M-mode and two-dimensional echocardiographic imaging with qualitative pulsed Doppler evaluations have been in widespread use for a number of years. With the current, ready availability of these techniques, complemented and supplemented with continuous wave Doppler (particularly with spatial orientation by color flow imaging), the performance of reliable *quantitative* Doppler echocardiography need not be confined to the research laboratory but can now be utilized very effectively in the clinical practice setting. The addition of Doppler techniques, after the standard M-mode and two-dimensional (2-D) echocardiographic examination, can add important additional diagnostic information in 60 to 70% of the patients studied.

In this book the term "quantitative" is being utilized for emphasis. Perhaps more appropriate terminology in some areas of the Doppler examination would be "semiquantitative." Full cognizance, however, is given to the fact that, by and large, medicine is an inexact science and contains few if any mathematically or physically precise "gold standards." The same comments apply even to data derived from cardiac catheterization studies. In many circumstances, Doppler-derived information may be "biologically" more precise and clinically more useful than catheter-determined data.

The goal of this book is to translate rather complex concepts and formulations into practical, easily understood and expeditiously applied evaluations which should allow any properly equipped echocardiographic laboratory to enjoy the rewards of quantitative cardiac Doppler. The information provided herein should be of greatest value to Cardiology Fellows in training and to practicing cardiologists who wish to upgrade the level of noninvasive diagnostic capabilities in their Doppler echocardiography laboratory.

THE AUTHOR

John H. Phillips, M.D., has been Professor of Medicine and Section Chief of Cardiology at Tulane University School of Medicine since 1973. In 1985, he was named the first Sidney W. and Marilyn S. Lassen Professor of Cardiovascular Medicine at Tulane. A native of Houston, Texas, Dr. Phillips earned his medical degree in 1955 from Tulane University School of Medicine. From 1956 to 1962, he served on the Tulane faculty. While at Tulane, Dr. Phillips interned at Charity Hospital of New Orleans and served as a National Heart Institute Research Fellow. Upon finishing his fellowship, he served with the U.S. Navy as Lt. Commander and Chief of the Cardiopulmonary Laboratories at the U.S. Navy as Lt. Commander and Chief of the Cardiopulmonary Laboratories at the U.S. Naval Hospital in Norfolk-Portsmouth, Virginia. In 1966, he returned to the Tulane faculty. Twice he has been named "Outstanding Teacher of the Year" by Tulane's Owl Club in addition to receiving the Gloria P. Walsh Award for Teaching Excellence. Dr. Phillips is a consultant in medicine and cardiology at many area hospitals and a Diplomate of the American Board of Internal Medicine and the Sub-specialty Board of Cardiovascular Disease. He is a Fellow and prior member of the Board of Trustees of the American College of Cardiology. He is also a Fellow of the American College of Chest Physicians, the American College of Physicians, and of the Council on Clinical Cardiology of the American Heart Association.

Throughout his career, Dr. Phillips has authored and/or co-authored over 150 scientific publications. His research interests have been in noninvasive cardiology, primarily electrocardiography and echocardiography.

ACKNOWLEDGMENTS

The senior author wishes to acknowlege the technical assistance of Ms. Jane Caire, B.S., the editorial assistance of Ms. Rebecca Levy, B.S. and the clerical assistance of Ms. Beth Lobell. The photography was provided by Mr. Robert Moldaner and the art work by Ms. Barbara Pendzimaz, B.S. Finally, for providing inspiration over the years, I acknowledge my close friends Dr. J. Karlem Riess, Dr. Robert D. Sparks and Mrs. Shirley Sparks, and my wife, Mary Jo, and children Virginia, Hunter, and Cynthia.

DEDICATION

This book is dedicated to Mr. Sidney W. Lassen and Mrs. Marilyn Sizeler Lassen, without whose generous support this work could not have been accomplished.

TABLE OF CONTENTS

Chapter 1

INTRODUCTION

The relatively complex fundamental basis of all the information to follow in the text of this book begins with the following:

$$\frac{\text{V max} = \text{C} \cdot \Delta f \text{ max}}{2 \cdot f_0 \cdot \cos \Theta} = \frac{1.54 \times \text{Doppler Shift (max)}}{2 \times \text{transducer frequency} \times \cos \Theta}$$

This is the *Doppler formula* where Vmax is the instantaneous maximum velocity of flow (cm/s), C is the velocity of sound in tissue (1.54×10^5 cm/s), Δf max is the instantaneous maximum frequency shift obtained from a spectrum analyzer (in Hz), f_0 is the frequency of the incident ultrasonic beam (in Hz) and cos Θ is the cosine of the angle between the axis of the transmitted ultrasonic beam and the direction of the maximum velocity vectors.

This monograph will assume that the reader has a working knowledge of the basic physics of Doppler technology and a practical understanding of the formula presented above. It is expected that the reader also has some prior experience with M-mode and 2-D echocardiography and with qualitative Doppler, particularly with reference to equipment operation and limitations, proper performance of the ultrasonic examinations, and accurate interpretation of the results. An understanding of Doppler terminology is helpful, including such terms (and techniques) as range-gating, aliasing (pulsed), gain settings, pulse repetition frequency (PRF), color-coded imaging, range ambiguity (CW), and ultrasonic beam angle of incidence dependency requirements. For a brief review of this pertinent echo-Doppler terminology, please consult the glossary.

The text of this book is organized in a manner whereby physical-physiological mechanisms and methods are presented first and then their practical applications are emphasized at various anatomic sites. Chapters 2, 3, and 4 deal basically with the most fundamental mechanisms wherein most of the evaluations of clinical relevance reside. These fundamental areas include pressure gradients, pressure half-times, and time velocity integrals. Once these "physiological" mechanisms are mastered, then the logical sequence is to approach the "anatomical" areas of the heart and great vessels. This is presented in an appropriate sequential fashion in the remaining text. Appendix A represents "technical tips" relative to the performance of the Doppler examination. The reader may wish to read this Appendix before pursuing the remainder of the book. Appendix B provides helpful blank "worksheets" and also worksheets completed with quantitative data from various valvular and hemodynamic abnormalities. Appendix C presents ready reference to normal and abnormal echo-Doppler values. The chapter summaries are presented in a manner which allows the reader a rapid review and recall of all the pertinent practical quantitative Doppler information presented in the chapter texts. These serve as a handy reference when the Doppler laboratory is presented specific problem areas for analysis.

The intent of this monograph is to impart information in the most expeditious and easily understood manner possible. In many instances, line drawings and artistic renditions accomplish this goal more readily than actual recordings. Although this may detract from the appeal of pristine originals, it much more readily allows the achievement of the goals of these presentations. Some "purists" may disagree, but those who wish to learn and apply the information practically will likely welcome this assistance and approach.

Chapter 2

PRESSURE GRADIENTS

I. INTRODUCTION

In the actively functioning cardiovascular system, pressure gradients (mmHg) are always present; these are what move the blood. In order to detect these gradients across cardiac valves by Doppler means, valvular "regurgitations" or "stenoses" must be present. Various published studies[1-4] reveal that regurgitations may be detected frequently even in normal hearts. The ranges in published series are tricuspid valve (15 to 95%), pulmonic valve (28 to 92%), mitral valve (10 to 45%) and aortic valve (0 to 33%). Valvular regurgitation and stenoses, of course, occur with increased frequency in diseased hearts, those most likely to warrant study. Therefore, Doppler pressure gradients can be determined in a large number of patients presenting for testing.

Once a maximum flow velocity (Vmax, m/s) across a valve (systole or diastole, regurgitation or stenosis) is recorded, then a pressure gradient across this valve can be readily determined using the Bernoulli equation.

The Bernoulli equation can be used to derive the pressure gradient in a pulsatile flow system. The equation is

$$\underbrace{P_1 - P_2}_{\substack{\text{pressure}\\ \text{gradient}}} = \underbrace{\tfrac{1}{2}\times r\left(V_2^2 - V_1^2\right)}_{\substack{\text{convective}\\ \text{acceleration}}} + \underbrace{r_1^2\,\frac{dv}{dt}\times ds}_{\substack{\text{flow}\\ \text{acceleration}}} + \underbrace{R(v)}_{\substack{\text{viscous}\\ \text{friction}\\ \text{loss}}}$$

Thus, three components influence the gradient: one for convective acceleration between the locations where V_1 and V_2 are measured (Figure 1); another for flow acceleration between the same locations; and lastly, one for the viscous friction loss between the same locations.

When using the simplified form of the Bernoulli equation, the following modifications are made: (1) at peak flow, the flow acceleration term is zero, (2) for the flow conditions in the heart and large vessels, the viscous friction loss is negligible, (3) assuming V_2 is much greater than V_1, then V_1 becomes negligible, and (4) using 1.07 g/cm^3 for ρ. Thus, the equation becomes

$$\Delta P = 4V^2$$

where ΔP is the pressure gradient and V is the distal (V_2) peak velocity.

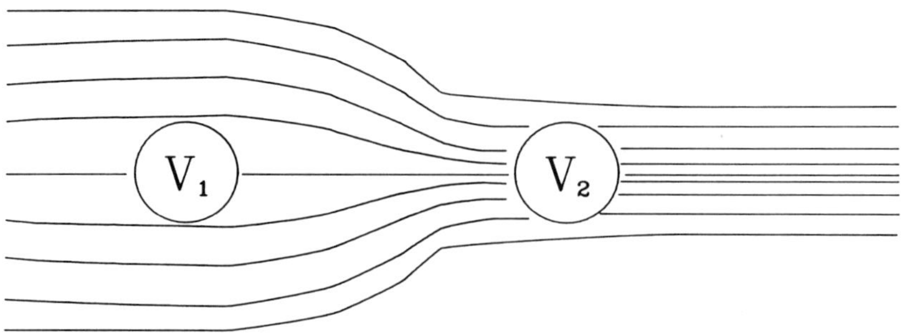

FIGURE 1. Illustrations of a flow system. The flow is in the direction of left to right and there is a "restriction" (stenosis) to flow between the area of V_1 and V_2. A *pressure gradient* develops between these two areas and for the same *volume of flow* to occur, the *velocity of flow* at V_2 must be much greater than the velocity flow at V_1.

In the vast majority of cases, particularly for clinical purposes, the shortened Bernoulli equation then may be utilized as:

$$G = 4V^2$$

where G is the gradient and V is the maximum instantaneous velocity (which is squared and multiplied by 4).

One may now proceed with the systematic study of valve gradients in both systole and diastole. The determined gradients then allow calculation of related pressures. The formulations which follow will denote those having *practical* application (i.e., in clinical studies) and those which are *theoretic* (their practical application not yet of utility primarily because of insufficient clinical correlations and/or technological limitations). It should be noted further that pressure determinations in association with the tricuspid valve (right-sided pressure) have been clinically validated whereas some of those pressure determinations on the left side of the heart require further study before they can be accepted with confidence.

II. SYSTOLIC GRADIENTS

A. PRACTICAL
l. Aortic Valve (aortic stenosis)

$$LV - AOR = G$$

where LV is peak systolic left ventricular pressure, AOR is peak systolic pressure in the aortic root and G is the peak systolic gradient across the stenotic

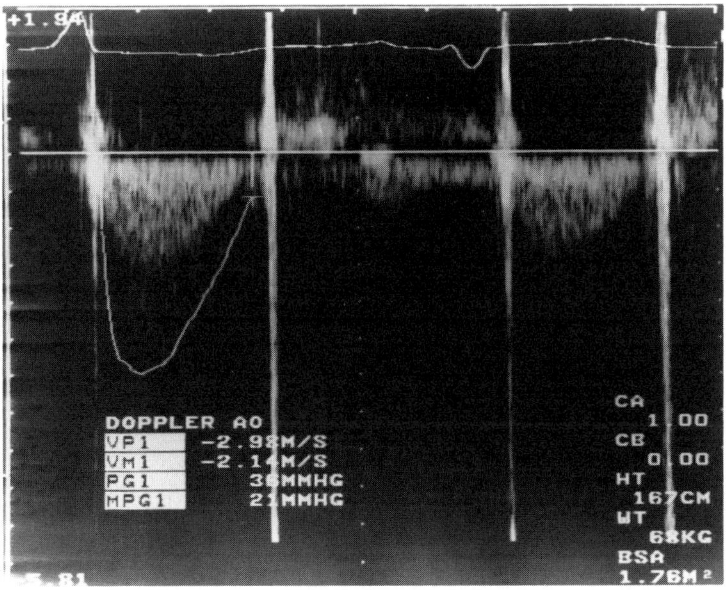

FIGURE 2. CW recording across left ventricular outflow tract (LVOT) from a patient with aortic stenosis. Vmax of 2.98 m/s noted and measured. Vertical calibration markers (velocity) = 0.5 m/s. Calculated G = 36 mmHg. With a systolic BP (cuff recorded) of 100 mmHg, the LV systolic pressure would then be 136 mmHg.

aortic valve (see also Chapter 4). This is one of the "gold standards" for aortic stenosis (AS) as might be determined at cardiac catheterization. For example, in mmHg, an LV of 140 with AOR of 100 would yield a G of 40. This formula may be rearranged for Doppler purposes as:

$$G + \text{AOR} = \text{LV systolic pressure}$$

where the G is determined from the CW maximum flow velocity ($4V^2$) and the AOR pressure is determined by clinical arm blood pressure (BP) cuff systolic pressure. For example (Figure 2), the recorded Vmax across the aortic valve is 2.98 m/s, the gradient ($4V^2$) is calculated [$4 \times (2.98)^2$] at 36 mmHg, the systolic BP is recorded as 100 mmHg, thus:

$$G\,(36) + \text{BP}\,(100) = \text{LV systolic pressure}\,(136)$$

The above calculation is of more practical importance in understanding the gradient concept than it is to clinical application. The calculation immediately following, however, is of considerable clinical value.

2. Tricuspid Valve (tricuspid regurgitation)

Since tricuspid regurgitation is a very common finding in cardiac Doppler, even in normal hearts, this formula is frequently utilized and yields extremely valuable data:

$$RV - RA = G$$

where RV is the right ventricular pressure, RA is the right atrial pressure, and G is the systolic pressure gradient across the tricuspid valve.

Rearranged:

$$G + RA = RV \text{ systolic } (\text{or PA systolic}) \text{ pressure } (\text{mmHg})$$

For example, G (20) + RA (5) = RV systolic pressure (25).

Since the RA pressure may be estimated at the bedside (e.g., jugular venous pulse) or at the Doppler examination (two methods to be described), the RV systolic pressure and, in the absence of pulmonic stenosis (PS), the pulmonary artery (PA) systolic pressure can be easily determined for most patients studied.

The RA pressure may be estimated at the Doppler exam by two methods. One method relates to the severity of tricuspid regurgitation (TR) usually determined by color flow mapping. Thus, one could add the RA to the G in the formula by the following estimates:

Trivial TR — add 5 mmHg RA
Mild TR — add 10 mmHg RA
Moderate TR — add 15 mmHg RA
Severe TR — add 20 mmHg RA

A more reliable method for estimating the RA pressure deals with determining the size ("congested" or not) of the inferior vena cava (IVC) and whether or not there is a decrease in size of the IVC during inspiration (or a "sniff"). The IVC values are as follows (determined from the 2-D imaging study, subxyphoid window, measured within 2 cm of IVC entrance to RA):

Nondilated <1.5 cm
Borderline 1.5 to 2.0 cm
Dilated >2.0 cm
Decrease with deep inspiration
Normal >50%
Abnormal <50%

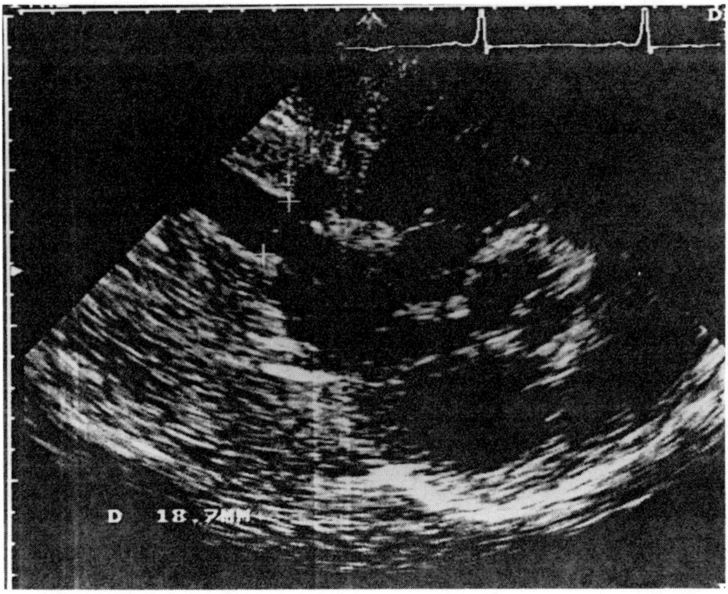

FIGURE 3. 2-D, subxyphoid view, IVC measured at entrance to RA, measured between markers (+) with a measurement of 1.87 cm. This is borderline dilated, thus allowing ann estimate of the RAP of 5 to 10 mmHg.

Thus, to estimate the RA pressure (RAP) and determine what needs to be added to G in the formula is as follows:

Nondilated — add 5 mmHg RA
Borderline — add 5 to 10 mmHg RA
Dilated but with normal inspiratory variation — add 10 to 15 mmHg RA
Dilated with abnormal inspiratory variation — add 15 to 20 mmHg RA

Figure 3 illustrates the measurement of IVC which gives an estimated RAP of 5 to 10 mmHg (average = 7).

Figure 4 is a continuous wave (CW) recording of the Vmax of a TR jet. The RV to RA gradient (G) is 23 mmHg. Therefore, 23 + 7 = 30 mmHg for the RV systolic pressure and the PA systolic pressure.

3. Ventricular Septal Defect

$$LV - RV = G$$

Rearranged:

$$LV - G = RV \text{ or PA systolic pressure}$$

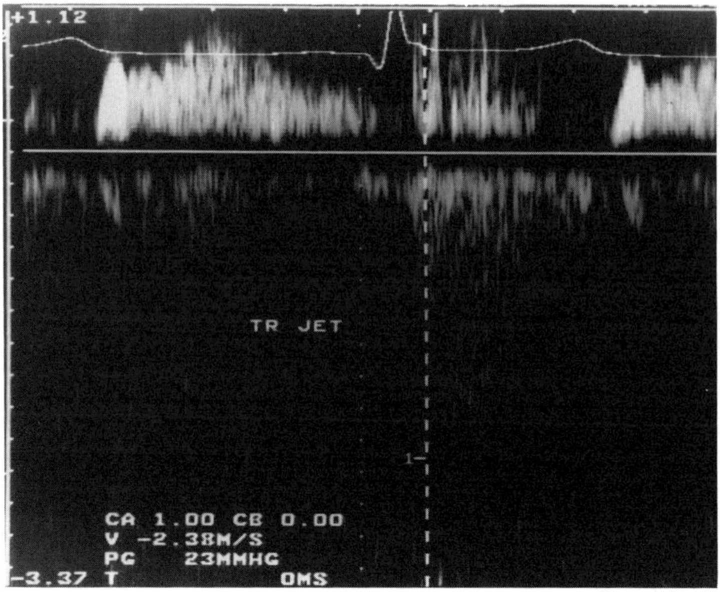

FIGURE 4. Color-Doppler-directed CW recording of Vmax in TR jet. Vertical calibration scale (velocity) each = 0.25 m/s. TR jet Vmax = 2.38 m/s measured at level "1". Calculated G = 23 mmHg.

where the LV is the systolic pressure (measured in arm with BP cuff, in absence of aortic stenosis), G is gradient ($4V^2$) measured across the ventricular septal defect (VSD), and RV and PA are the RV systolic and PA systolic pressures (in absence of PS).

4. Mitral Valve (mitral regurgitation)

Technical limitations may render this determination inaccurate and thus care should be given in its clinical application.

$$LV - LA = G$$

Rearranged:

$$LV\ (\text{BP cuff, absence of AS}) - G = LA$$

$$LA \propto PCW \propto PA\ \text{diastolic}$$

B. THEORETIC

The following is a theoretic formulation. It is presented basically for interest and completeness.

1. Pulmonic Valve (pulmonic stenosis)

$$RV - PA = G$$

Rearranged:

$$RV\ (\text{formula from Section II.A.2}) - G = PA \text{ systolic pressure}$$

In pulmonic stenosis, since the measurement of most clinical importance is the gradient (G) across the pulmonic valve (measured as $4V^2$), this formula, as noted, is largely of theoretic interest only.

III. DIASTOLIC GRADIENTS

A. PRACTICAL

l. Aortic valve (aortic valvular insufficiency)

$$AOR - LV = G$$

Rearranged:

$$AOR - G = LVEDP$$

where AOR is diastole pressure measured in the arm by cuff method, G is the end-diastolic gradient ($4V^2$) of the velocity (measured at the end of the slope of the aortic insufficiency spectral flow pattern) and LVEDP is the LV end diastolic pressure.

Figure 5 is a CW recording of an aortic insufficiency (AI) spectral display revealing an end-diastolic gradient of 49 mmHg. With an arm BP cuff-recorded diastolic pressure of 60 mmHg, the LVEDP would be 11 mmHg ($60 - 49 = 11$).

2. Pulmonic Valve (pulmonic valve insufficiency)

$$PA - RV = G$$

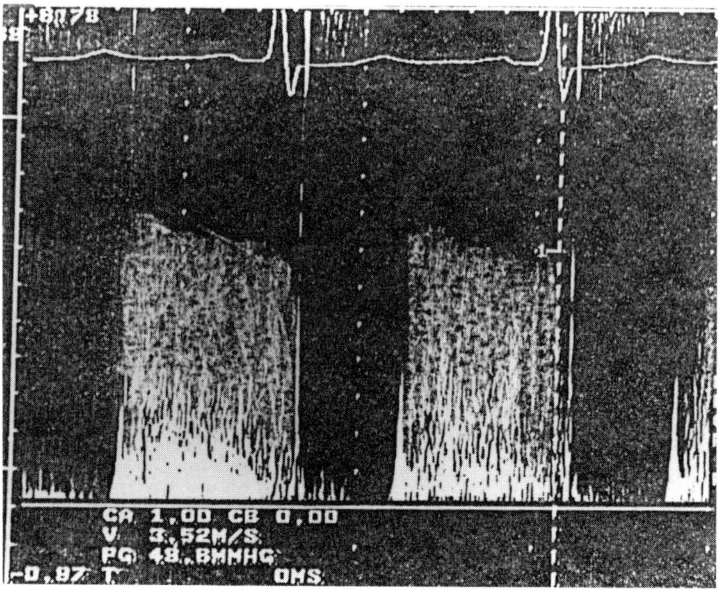

FIGURE 5. CW recording (apical 4 chamber view) of AI spectral display (artistically retouched for clarity). Vertical calibrations each as 0.5 m/s. Velocity of AI at end diastolic = 3.52 m/s (measured at point "1"). Thus, the end diastolic aortic to LV gradient is approximately 49 mmHg. The cuff recorded BP was 158/60. Thus, 60 – 49 = 11 mmHg for the LVEDP.

When PA is the diastolic pressure in the PA, RV is the diastolic pressure in the RV (estimated from RA diastolic at 5 mmHg) and G is the end-diastolic gradient ($4V^2$) of the velocity measured at the end of the slope of the pulmonic insufficiency spectral flow pattern.

Rearranged:

$$RV + G = PA \text{ diastolic pressure}$$

$$RV \text{ diastolic} = \text{estimated RA diastolic (usually approximates 5 mmHg)}$$

$$(PA \text{ diastolic} \propto \text{pulmonary capillary wedge} \propto LVEDP.$$

Figure 6 is a spectral display of a pulmonic valve insufficiency (PI) jet (CW recording). The PA to RV end-diastolic gradient is 4.5 mmHg. Assuming an RVEDP of 5 mmHg, then the PA diastolic pressure would be 9.5 mmHg.

B. THEORETIC

Again, these are presented primarily for interest and completeness. They may prove of practical value in some situations, however.

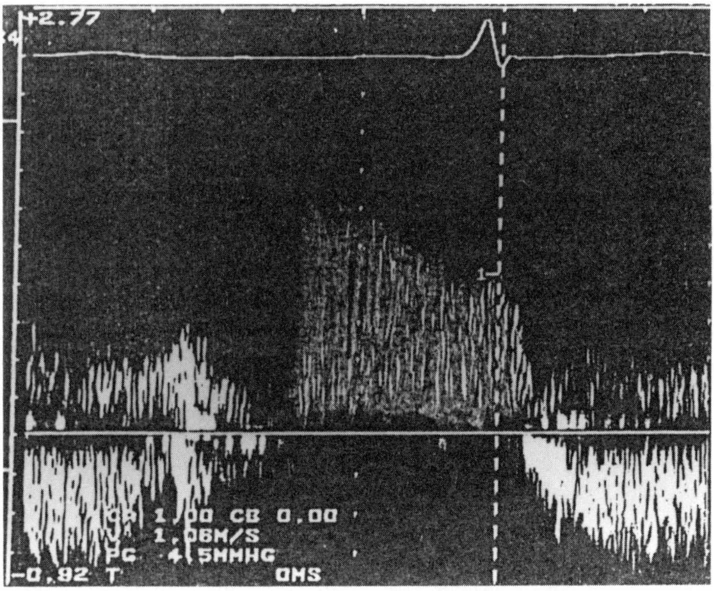

FIGURE 6. CW recording (parasternal short axis, PA level) of a PI jet. Vertical calibration each at 0.25 m/s. Velocity of PI at end diastolic = 1.06 m/s (measured at point "1"). Thus, the end diastolic PA to RV gradient is 4.5 mmHg. Assuming an RVEDP of 5 mmHg, then 4.5 + 5 = 9.5 mmHg for PA diastolic pressure. This pressure, of course, approximates the pulmonary capillary wedge pressure and the LVEDP. The figure is artistically slightly retouched for clarity.

1. Mitral Valve (mitral stenosis)

$$LA - LV = G$$

The gradient, of course, is of the most clinical value in this formula. Rearranged:

$$LA \text{ (formula from Section II. A. 4)} - G = LVEDP$$

2. Tricuspid Valve (tricuspid stenosis)

$$RA - RV = G$$

Rearranged:

$$RA - G = RVEDP$$

where RVEDP = RV end-diastolic pressure.

As Doppler technology advances, allowing for detection and accurate definition of even minor degrees of regurgitation and stenosis, the above formulations (even those now of only theoretic interest) may achieve increasing clinical importance. These determinations will then allow the serial noninvasive evaluation of intravascular pressures. This will prove of great value in the delineation of the natural history of certain diseases and in the response of various diseases to differing forms of therapy (both acute and chronic).

IV. SUMMARY

"Gradients" are based on the presence of stenoses or regurgitations. Regurgitations are present normally as:

TR — 15 to 95%
PR — 28 to 92%
MR — 10 to 45%
AR — 0 to 33%

Gradients and related pressure calculations of clinical value during *systole* are

Aortic valve (AS)
  LV − AOR = G
  G + AOR (BP cuff) = LV systolic pressure
Tricuspid valve (TR)
  RV − RA = G
  G + RA = RV systolic (= PAP) pressure
IVC measurements
  Nondilated <1.5 cm
  Borderline 1.5 to 2.0 cm
  Dilated >2.0 cm
  Decrease with deep inspiration
    Normal >50%
    Abnormal <50%
Estimate RA by IVC
  Nondilated — add 5 mmHg
  Borderline — add 5 to 10 mmHg
  Dilated but with normal inspiratory variation, add 10 to 15 mmHg
  Dilated with abnormal inspiratory variation, add 15 to 20 mmHg

Gradients and related pressure calculations of clinical value during *diastole* are

Aortic valve (AI)
AOR – LV = G (end diastole)
AOR (BP cuff, diastolic) – G = LVEDP

REFERENCES

1. **Yoshida, K., et al.,** Color Doppler evaluation of valvular regurgitation in normal subjects, *Circulation,* 78, 840, 1988.
2. **Yoch, P.G., Schnittger, I., and Popp, R.L.,** Is continuous wave Doppler too sensitive in diagnosing pathologic valvular regurgitation (Abstract), *Circulation,* 70 (Suppl. 2), 381, 1984.
3. **Kostucki, W., Vandenbossche, J., Friart, A., and Englert, M.,** Pulsed Doppler regurgitant flow patterns in normal valves, *Am. J. Cardiol.,* 58, 309, 1986.
4. **Sahn, D.J. and Maciel, B.C.,** Physiological valvular regurgitation, *Circulation,* 78, 1075, 1988.

ADDITIONAL READING

Yoganathan, A.P., et al., Review of hemodynamic principles for the cardiologist: applications to the study of blood flow and jets by imaging techniques, *J. Am. Coll. Cardiol.,* 12, 1344, 1988.

Cooper, J.W., Nanda, N.C., Philpot, E.F., and Fan, P., Evaluation of valvular regurgitation by color Doppler, *J. Am. Soc. Echocardiol.,* 2, 56, 1989.

Moreno, F.L., et al., Evaluation of size and dynamics of the inferior vena cava as an index of right-sided cardiac function, *Am. J. Cardiol.,* 53, 579, 1984.

Yock, P.G. and Popp, R.L., Non-invasive estimation of right ventricular systolic pressure by Doppler ultrasound in patients with tricuspid regurgitation, *Circulation,* 70, 657, 1984.

Simonson, J.S. and Schiller, N.B., Sonospirometry: a new method for noninvasive estimation of mean right atrial pressure based on two dimensional echocardiographic measurements of the inferior vena cava during measured inspiration, *J. Am. Coll. Cardiol.,* 11, 557, 1988

Chapter 3

PRESSURE HALF-TIMES

I. DISCUSSION

Pressure half-times (P1/2t) may be determined wherever pressure gradients (see Chapter 2) can be recorded. P1/2t has displayed its greatest utility in relation to transmitral diastolic flow in the presence of mitral stenosis (see Chapter 6), and, thus, this model serves best for discussion of the P1/2t concept and formulations. Since changes in pressure gradients are exponential over time, then the graphic displays of these relationships are usually presented on semilogarithmic paper with the pressure gradient (mmHg) shown on the ordinate and the time (ms) shown on the abscissa (presented diagrammatically in Figure 1). Note in example "A" the peak gradient is 30 mmHg. The decline in the gradient to 1/2 of this value (15 mmHg) takes approximately 230 ms, this then being the P1/2t. In example "B," the peak gradient is 20 mmHg. The decline in the gradient to 1/2 of this value (10 mmHg) takes approximately 360 ms, the P1/2t for this example. As will be seen, the P1/2t provides a valuable index of the severity of mitral stenosis.

It has been shown that the relationship between velocity (m/s) and pressure gradient (mmHg) is quadratic.[1] Therefore, the pressure half-time may be calculated by dividing the initial peak velocity by $\sqrt{2}$ (or 1.41) and measuring the time taken for the peak velocity to decline to the latter level (P1/2t). As presented diagrammatically in Figure 2, the Doppler determined velocity (m/s) is not plotted on semilog paper (thus, the need to divide by $\sqrt{2}$ when comparing to semilog, displayed pressure gradient, ordinate). In this figure the early instantaneous peak velocity (Vmax) is displayed as 2 m/s, giving a gradient ($4V^2$) at this point of 16 mmHg. Note that one could then calculate the instantaneous gradients anywhere along the flow velocity curve, determining the mean gradient and even the end-diastolic gradient (elevated, of course, in mitral stenosis). The P1/2t in mitral stenosis is a better gauge of hemodynamic alteration than end-diastolic gradients, however, since this time is not influenced significantly by changes in cycle length (e.g., virtually no gradient at the end of a very long diastolic period), cardiac output, or the presence of mitral regurgitation. It may not be accurate in the presence of severe aortic regurgitation (see Chapter 6 for details).

Thus, as presented in Figure 2, the early diastolic peak mitral flow velocity (Vmax) is measured (2 m/s) and divided by $\sqrt{2}$ (or divided by 1.4 or multiplied by 0.71, all mathematical equivalents) to obtain the *velocity* at which *time* the *pressure* gradient has fallen to one half of the peak pressure. Then, the *time*

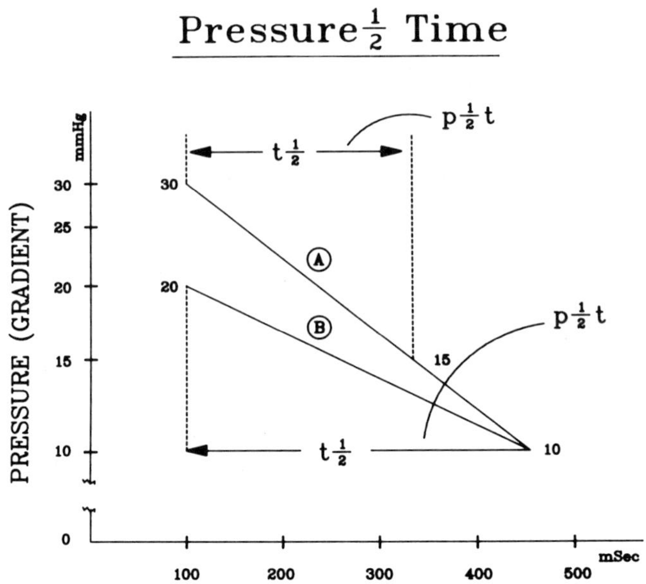

FIGURE 1. Pressure half-times, examples "A" and "B". Please consult text for details.

required for the peak *velocity* to fall to the *velocity corresponding* to *one half of the peak pressure* is measured in milliseconds (ms) and recorded then as the P1/2t. Thus, in the example given,

$$\frac{\text{V max}}{\sqrt{2}} = \frac{2}{1.4} = 1.43\text{m m / s}$$

and the time for the Vmax to fall to this level would be the P1/2t (approximately 100 ms in the example given). It was found[2] that in mitral stenosis the mitral valve area (MVA) could be estimated from the P1/2t by the formula:

$$\text{MVA}\left(\text{cm}^2\right) = \frac{220}{\text{P1/2t (m / s)}}$$

Thus, a P1/2t of 220 would be equivalent to a MVA of 1 cm^2 (see Chapter 6 for details).

Figure 3 illustrates a PW Doppler-recorded mitral diastolic flow pattern from a normal patient (vertical velocity calibrations at 0.05 m/s). The early peak diastolic flow velocity (Vmax) = 0.99 m/s.

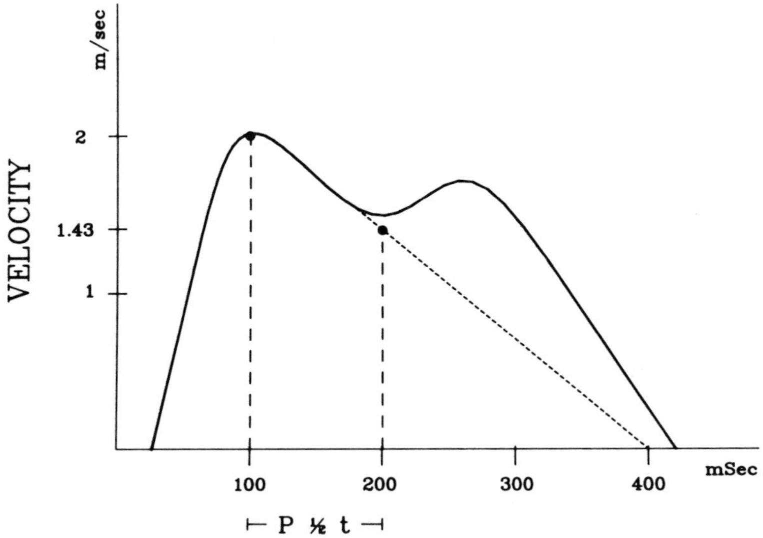

FIGURE 2. Diagrammatic representation of transmitral diastolic flow velocity. Vmax = 2.0 m/s.

$$\frac{\text{V max}}{\sqrt{2}} = \frac{2}{1.4} = 1.43 \text{ m/s}$$

The time for the Vmax to fall to 1.43 m/s = P1/2t or, in this example, about 100 ms.

The time required for the Vmax to fall to 0.7 m/s is 42 ms = P1/2t. Normal mitral P1/2t = 20 – 60 m/s. In the example given:

$$\text{MVA} = \frac{220}{42} = 5.24 \text{ cm}^2$$

Normal MVA area = 4 to 6 cm.[2]

An alternate method for determining the mitral diastolic P1/2t utilizes the following formula:[3]

$$0.29 \times \text{Deceleration time} = \text{P 1/2t}$$

See Chapter 6 for further information relative to the above.

II. SUMMARY

Pressure half-time (P1/2t) may be calculated as follows:

$$\frac{\text{V max}}{\sqrt{2}} = \frac{\text{V max}}{1.4} = \begin{array}{c}\text{The } \textit{velocity} \text{ fall} \\ \text{from Vmax}\end{array}$$

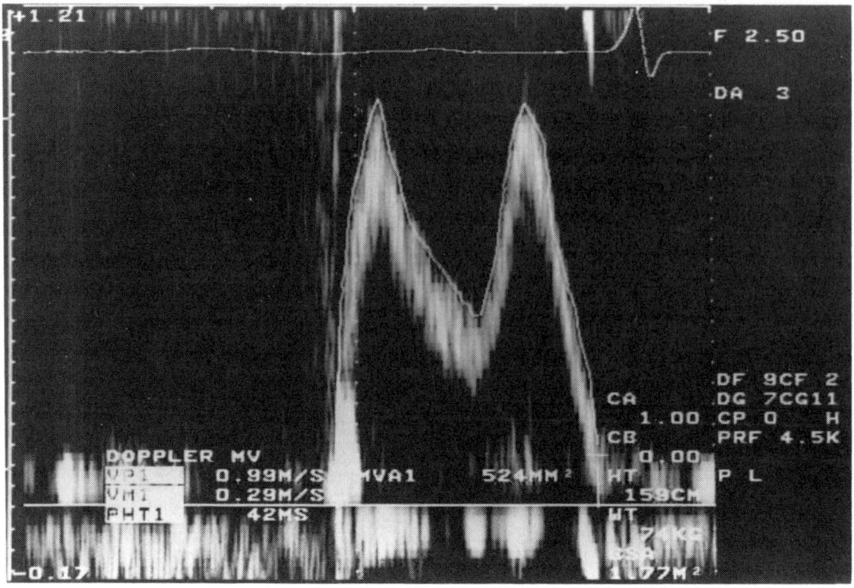

FIGURE 3. PW Doppler-recorded transmitral diastolic flow pattern from a normal patient. The early Vmax = 0.99 m/s

$$\frac{V\,\max}{\sqrt{2}} = \frac{0.99}{1.4} = 0.7\ \text{m/s}$$

The time taken for V max to fall to 0.7 m/s = 42 m/s = P1/2t. (Calculations are also provided automatically by equipment computer program, note the print-out numbers on the illustration). Horizontal time lines (at top) represent 100 ms each.

which would be equivalent in *time* occurrence to that of a *pressure* gradient which would have fallen to one half (P1/2t).

Alternatively, 0.29 × Deceleration time = P1/2t.

REFERENCES

1. **Hatle, L. and Angelsen, B.,** *Doppler ultrasound in cardiology,* Lea & Febiger, Philadelphia, 1982
2. **Hatle, L., Angelsen, B., and Tromsdal, A.,** Non-invasive assessment of atrioventricular pressure half-time by Doppler ultrasound, *Circulation,* 60, 1096, 1979.
3. **Pearlman, J. D. and Gibson, R.,** Doppler measurement of left atrial depressurization and mitral valve area in patients with suspected mitral stenosis: validation of a new method, *Am. Heart J.,* 113, 868, 1987.

Chapter 4

TIME VELOCITY INTEGRALS

I. DISCUSSION

The time velocity integral (TVI) concept and related formulations have proven of great benefit in quantitative Doppler echocardiography, specifically in determining stroke volumes and cardiac output. The TVI has been used interchangeably with time velocity index, flow velocity integral (FVI) and flow velocity index. The TVI represents the *integration* of the Doppler flow velocity curve. The *units* for the TVI are *centimeters* (cm) (Figure 1).

Flow (F or Q) or cardiac output (CO) is essentially *volume* (V) or stroke volumes (SV) moved *per unit of time* (t) or heart beats at a given heart rate (bpm), (Figure 2). *Volume* (V in cm^3) may be calculated by multiplying *area* (cm^2) by *length* (cm), (Figure 3):

$$V\left(cc \text{ or } cm^3\right) = A\left(cm^2\right) \times L(cm)$$

Area (A) may be easily calculated knowing the diameter (d) of the structure studied (e.g., the left ventricular outflow tract, aortic root, or the pulmonary artery), (Figure 4):

$$A = \pi\, r^2 = 3.14\left(\frac{d}{2}\right)^2 = cm^2$$

Length (L in cm) is the distance over which the volume flows per unit of time and is derived from the TVI (unit = cm) (Figure 5). If one knows the *velocity* (cm/s) at which a volume moves and over what *time* period (s) this volume moves, then one can easily calculate the *length* (cm) or distance moved. Relative to the TVI, consider the example of a red cell moving at a mean velocity (average speed) of 50 cm/s for one-half second (time). The distance (length) moved would then be 25 cm during that given period of time.

The integration of the flow velocity curve (Figure 1) can be derived by planimetry or by multiplying the mean velocity of the curve by the ejection time (ET) (Figure 6):

$$TVI = \text{Mean Vel} \times ET = L$$

Thereby, the length (L) in centimeters ("stroke distance") is derived. Thus,

$$Vol = A \times L$$

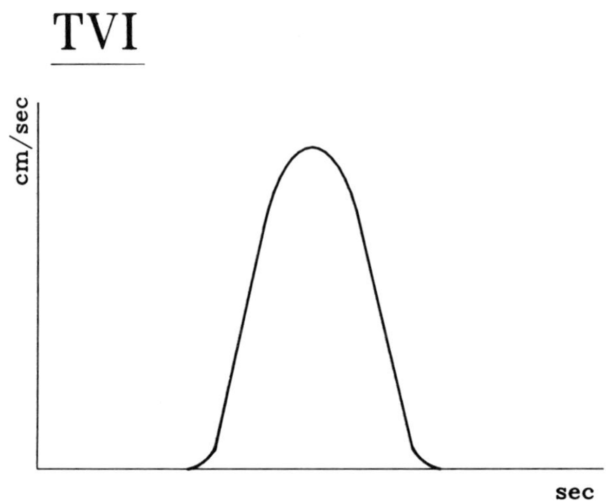

$$TVI = \frac{cm \times sec}{sec} = cm$$

FIGURE 1. Diagrammatic representation of a flow velocity curve. In this example, the velocity (ordinate or y axis) is presented in cm/s and the time (abscissa or x axis) is presented in seconds (s). It is clear that the integration of this curve gives units which are in centimeters (cm) (length or distance).

The "unknown" is the volume or volume moved (Figure 7). The area (A) of specific interest may be determined by the M-mode and/or 2-D Echo image study. The length (L) may be determined by Doppler velocity study (e.g., the mean velocity at which the volume moved and the time over which this volume moved = TVI) (Figure 7). Thus, SV may be calculated (Figure 8):

$$SV(\text{cc or cm}^3) = A(\text{cm}^2) \times L(\text{cm})$$

Recall that flow (F) is volume (V) moved per unit of time (e.g., seconds) and therefore flow (cm^3/s) equals the velocity (Vel) of flow (e.g., cm/s) times the area (A) of flow (cm^2) (Figure 9).

Thus, CO may be calculated as (Figure 10):

$$Q = \text{Flow}(F) = CO = SV \times HR = 1/\text{min}$$

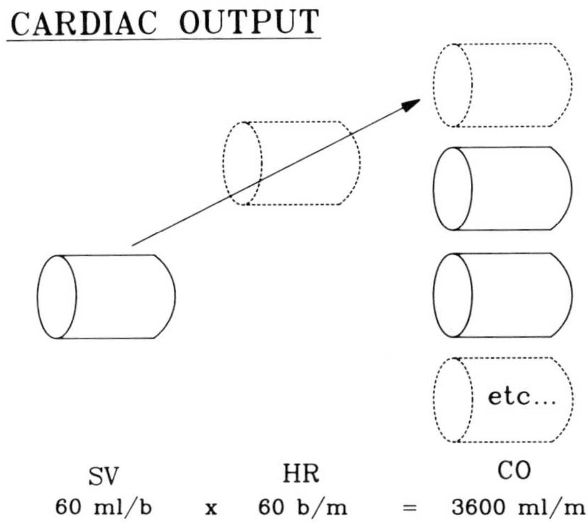

FIGURE 2. The stroke volume (SV) moved with a single beat may be visualized as a "small can of blood". If each SV with each heart beat contains 60 ml of blood, and if the heart rate is 60 bpm, then 3600 ml (60×60) would be the volume of blood moved in 1 min., i.e., cardiac output (CO) = 3600 ml/min or 3.6 l/min.

Please consult Chapters 5 and 9 for details of the *practical application* of the concepts presented here.

The various relationships of area, distance, time, and volume moved can be easily appreciated (Figure 11). When the volume (V) moved and time (ET) moved are kept constant, then, if the area (A) increases, the velocity (V, cm/s) decreases; whereas, if the area (A) decreases, then the velocity (V, cm/s) increases.

Where technical or time-limitation problems cause difficulty in the above (e.g., calculation of mean velocity), the TVI may be estimated by the following equation:

$$\text{TVI} = \frac{\text{PV} \times \text{ET}}{2} = \text{cm}$$

where PV is the peak velocity in cm/s and ET is the ejection time in seconds. Since this equation usually underestimates the true TVI, it should be recognized as only an estimate.

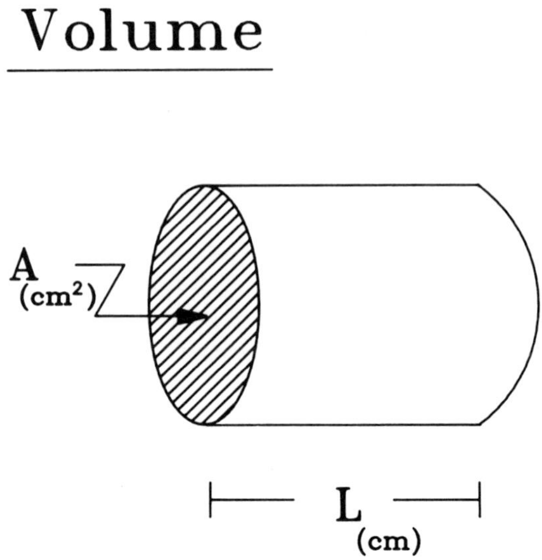

FIGURE 3. Volume (V) of a "container" is calculated by

$$V = \text{area (A)} \times \text{length (L)}$$

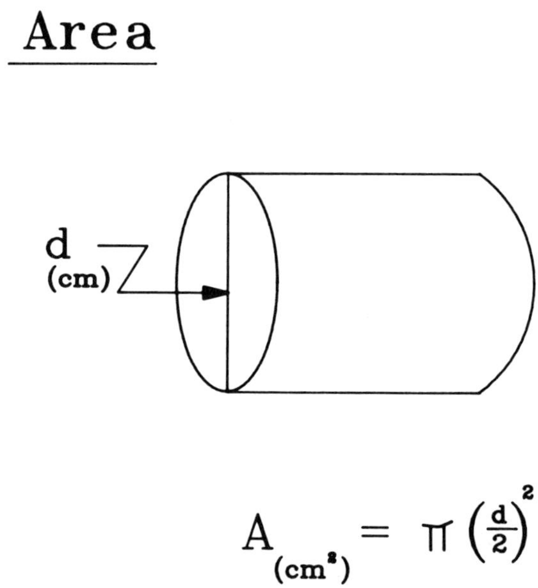

FIGURE 4. The area (A) of a circular plane is calculated by

$$A\left(\text{cm}^3\right) = \left(\frac{d}{2}\right)^2 = \pi r^2$$

where d is the diameter of the circle, r is the radius, and π is 3.1416.

Length

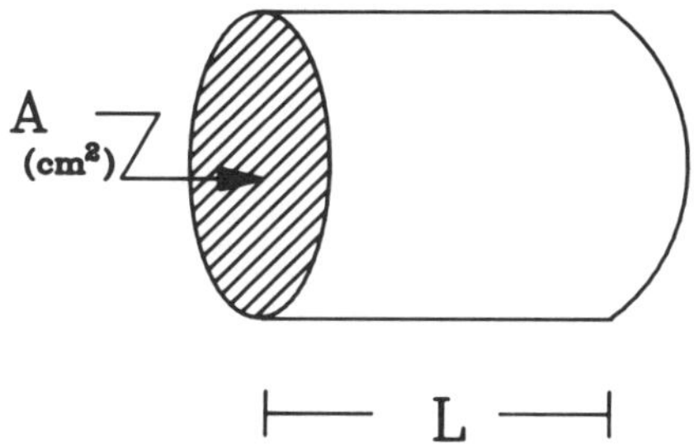

$$L = TVI = \frac{cm \times sec}{sec} = cm$$

FIGURE 5. Length (L in cm) is the distance over which movement occurs. If one determines the velocity of movement (cm/s) and the time (s) of movement, the distance moved (length) is then easily calculated.

Time Velocity Integral (TVI)

$$TVI = \text{Mean Velocity} \times ET$$

$$TVI = \frac{cm}{\cancel{sec}} \times \cancel{sec} = cm$$

FIGURE 6. A flow velocity curve is presented in Figure 1. Here, the ejection time (ET) is the time (s) from the onset to the end of the curve. The peak of the curve is the maximum velocity (Vmax). By hand calculation, multiple time points along the velocity curve may be measured, then averaged, thus deriving the mean velocity. The computer package of modern equipment automatically provides both the peak and the mean velocity and, thus, time-consuming hand-derived methods are unnecessary. As illustrated in Figure 6, multiplying the mean velocity (cm/s) by the ET (s) results in the TVI or length (distance) moved (cm).

Volume / Volume Moved

Unknown ⟶ V or V moved

M / 2D ⟶ A ⟶ Area moved through

Doppler ⟶ L ⟶ { Velocity at which moved and Time of movement or TVI.

FIGURE 7. Volume/volume moved. Consult text for details.

Stroke Volume (SV)

$$\underset{(\text{cc or cm}^3)}{SV} = \underset{(\text{cm}^2)}{A} \times \underset{(\text{cm})}{L}$$

FIGURE 8. Calculation of stroke volume (SV). A = area (of chamber through which volume moves). L = length or the distance moved.

II. SUMMARY

The time velocity integral (TVI) is important in the calculations of volumes (V) and flows (Q).

$$L_{cm} = TVI = \text{mean velocity} \times ET = cm$$

$$A_{cm^2} = \pi r^2 = cm^2$$

$$V_{cm^3} = A_{cm^2} \times L_{cm}$$

$$SV_{cm^3} = A_{cm^2} \times TVI$$

$$Q = CO = SV_{cm^3} \times HR = L/min$$

where A is area, L is length, r is radius of the structure through which flow occurs, ET is ejection time, SV is stroke volume, CO is cardiac output, HR is heart rate, and 1/min is liters per minute.

$$\underline{\text{Flow (F)} = \text{V per time}}$$

$$F = Vel \times A$$

$$\frac{cm^3}{sec} = \frac{cm}{sec} \times cm^2$$

FIGURE 9. Calculation of flow. Consult text for details.

Cardiac Output (CO)

$$\underset{(cm^3)}{SV} = \underset{(cm^2)}{A} \times \underset{(cm)}{L} = \underset{(cm^2)}{A} \times \underset{(cm)}{TVI}$$

$$F\ (Flow)_{\frac{cm^3}{sec}} = A_{cm^2} \times Vel_{\frac{cm}{sec}}$$

$$\underset{\left(\frac{cm^3}{sec}\right)}{F\ (Flow)} = \underset{\left(\frac{cm^3}{stroke}\right)}{SV} \times \underset{\left(\frac{stroke(s)}{sec}\right)}{\#\text{ of Strokes per time}}$$

By substituting SV units with $\frac{\text{liter(s)}}{\text{heartbeat}}$ and number of strokes per time with $\frac{\text{heartbeat(s)}}{\text{min}}$ which is the heartrate.

Then: $Q = Flow(F) = CO = SV \times HR$

$$\underset{\left(\frac{liter(s)}{min}\right)}{CO} = \underset{\left(\frac{liter(s)}{heartbeat}\right)}{SV} \times \underset{\left(\frac{heartbeat(s)}{min}\right)}{HR} = L/min$$

$$\begin{aligned} CO &= TVI \times A \times HR \\ &= L \times A \times HR \\ &= \text{Mean Velocity} \times ET \times A \times HR \end{aligned}$$

FIGURE 10. Doppler calculation of cardiac output. Stroke volume (calculated as TVI × A) multiplied by the number of stroke volumes (heart beats) per minute provides the cardiac output (CO).

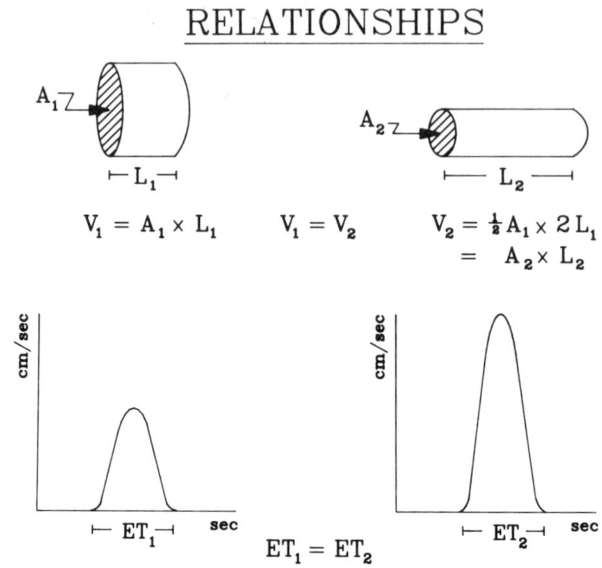

FIGURE 11. Relationships between area, distance, time, and volume moved. Where the volume moved is constant ($V_1 = V_2$) and the time (ET) over which this volume moves is constant, then, if the area through which this volume must move is reduced, then the velocity with which this volume moves must increase (and vice versa). In the examples given, note that the volumes are equal ($V_1 = V_2$) and the times moved or ET are equal ($ET_1 = ET_2$). The differences in the velocity curves are obvious.

ADDITIONAL READING

Lewis, J. F., et al., Pulsed Doppler echocardiographic determination of stroke volume and cardiac output: clinical validation of two new methods using the apical window, *Circulation,* 70, 425,1984.

Huntsman, L. L., et al., Non-invasive Doppler determination of cardiac output in man: clinical validation, *Circulation,* 60, 593, 1983.

Donnerstein, R. L. and Marx, G. R., A simplified method for determining Doppler velocity areas for cardiac output calculation, . *Circulation,* (Abstr.), 1987.

Nishimura, R. A., et al., Non-invasive measurement of cardiac output by continuous-wave Doppler echocardiography: initial experience and review of the literature, *Mayo Clin. Proc.,* 59, 484, 1984.

Chapter 5

AORTIC VALVE, AORTIC ROOT, AND LEFT VENTRICULAR OUTFLOW TRACT

I. INTRODUCTION

In the adult, the normal maximal flow velocity (Vmax) across the left ventricular outflow tract and aortic valve is less than 1.9 m/s. Normally, aortic stenosis is absent and theoretically, therefore, there should be no systolic flow gradient detected by Doppler examination across this area. Due to high flow velocities, small gradients (e.g., 5 to 10 or even 15 mmHg peak) are not infrequently recorded in normal subjects, however. Generally, Doppler examination reveals no aortic regurgitation in normals,[1] although "physiologic" regurgitation has been detected in up to 33% in one study.[2]

II. AORTIC STENOSIS (AS)

A. GRADIENTS ACROSS THE AORTIC VALVE

Gradients across the aortic valve represent one of the most common means of expressing the hemodynamic severity of aortic stenosis. These include the instantaneous gradient, the "peak to peak" gradient (commonly used in data obtained from cardiac catheterization), and the mean gradient (sum of all the instantaneous gradients divided by the ejection time). These various gradients are diagrammatically depicted in Figures 1 and 2. Although in very common use clinically, the "peak to peak" gradient is clearly not physiologic since the LV pressure (earlier peak) and aortic root pressure (later peak) do not coincide temporally.

The flow velocity curves across the LV outflow tract (LVOT), the aortic valve, and the aortic root can be easily recorded in most patients (Figure 3). Since flow velocities in this area are usually high, pulsed Doppler recordings frequently result in aliasing. Continuous wave (CW) Doppler is therefore usually employed. With proper technique (echo beam as parallel to flow as possible, 2-D, color flow, and/or audio signal directed) the Vmax is obtained. Utilizing the formula $4V^2$, the maximum instantaneous gradient is calculated (Figure 3). The mean velocity may be obtained by integrating the flow velocity curve (this calculation is usually provided in the computer software programs of most modern equipment). From the mean velocity, again utilizing $4V^2$, the mean gradient is obtained. This mean gradient approximates closely the peak to peak gradient recorded at cardiac catheterization (with gradients >50 mmHg usually indicating severe aortic stenosis). Discrepancies of any significance (i.e., catheter-determined peak to peak higher than the Doppler-determined mean gradient) occur only when very high gradients are present (e.g., >75 mmHg as determined by catheter).

Severity of Aortic Stenosis (Mean Gradient, mmHg):

Mild	<20
Moderate	20–50
Severe	>50

For given valve areas, pressure gradients vary directly with changes in cardiac output (CO) or stroke volume (SV). For this reason the calculation of aortic valve area utilizing the continuity equation has become popular.

B. CONTINUITY EQUATION

According to the *continuity equation,* when there is a constant flow in a flow channel with a stenosis, the flow volume at the stenotic portion equals that at the nonstenotic portions. This equation is valid not only in a constant flow channel, but also in a pulsatile flow channel, like the heart, if the time for observation is one cardiac cycle. Thus,

$$SV_1 = SV_2$$

where SV_1 is the stroke volume in the nonstenotic area (LVOT) and SV_2 is the stroke volume in the stenotic area (aortic valve). As discussed in detail in Chapter 4 the formulations are

$$SV = A\left(cm^2\right) \times L(cm)$$

$$A = \pi\, r^2 = cm^2$$

$$L = TVI = cm$$

$$TVI = \text{mean velocity} \times ET$$

where SV is stroke volume, A is area in cm^2, L is length in cm, radius is one-half diameter (of LVOT), TVI is the time velocity integral, and ET is the ejection time. Thus,

$$\frac{LVOT}{SV_1} = \frac{\text{Aortic valve}}{SV_2}$$

$$A_1 \times TVI_1 = A_2 \times TVI_2$$

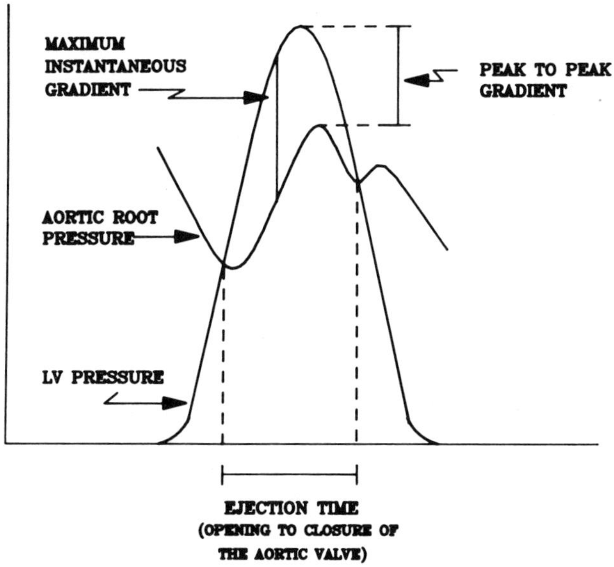

FIGURE 1. Aortic gradients illustrating the differences between maximum instantaneous gradient (generally derived by Doppler) and the peak to peak gradient (generally derived by cardiac catheterization).

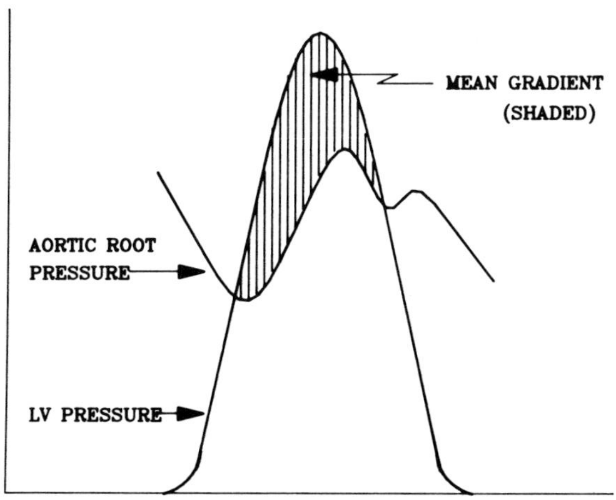

FIGURE 2. Mean aortic gradient. Compare this to the maximum gradient and the peak to peak gradient illustrated in Figure 1.

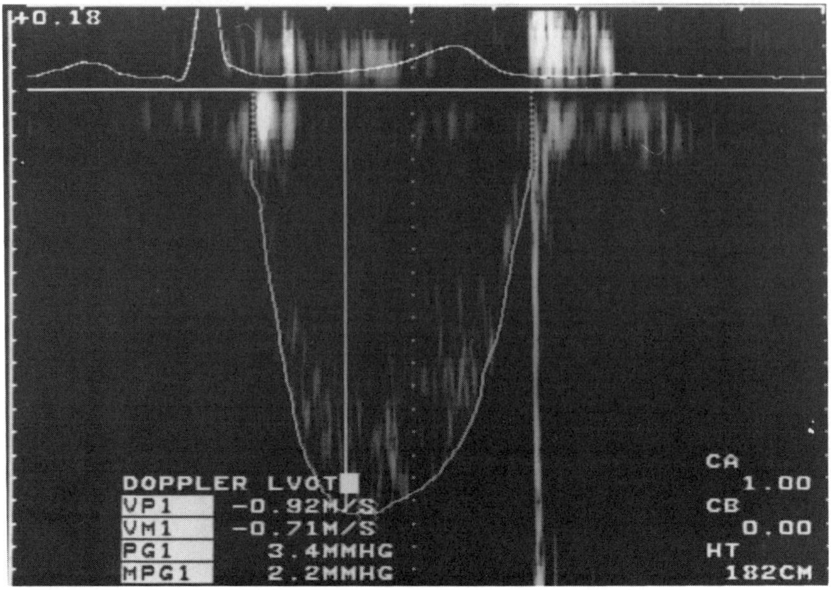

FIGURE 3. Normal LVOT systolic flow velocity curve. Vertical velocity calibrations are 0.05 m/s. Note LVOT peak velocity (Vmax) recorded at 0.92 m/s (normal is less than 1.9 m/s). The equipment software automatically calculates (integration) the mean velocity at 0.71 m/s. The maximum instantaneous gradient (peak gradient) is also provided automatically, or may be calculated ($4V^2 = 4 \times 0.92^2 = 3.4$ mmHg). The mean gradient is 2.2 mmHg.

Since the ET across the LVOT and the aortic valve are equivalent, the ET may be dropped from the equation. Since it is the *ratio* of velocities that is important, then the Vmax may be used instead of the mean velocity. Thus the TVI need not be calculated and Vmax (V_1 is the Vmax in the LVOT and V_2 is the Vmax across the aortic valve) may be substituted in the equation. Note that changes in systolic stroke volume would have equivalent effects on V_1 and V_2. The simplified formula then is

$$V_1 \times \text{LVOT area} = V_2 \times \text{AVA}$$

where AVA is the aortic valve area.

Rearranged:

$$\text{AVA}\left(\text{cm}^2\right) = \text{LVOT area}\left(\text{cm}^2\right) \times \frac{V_1 \ (\text{LVOT})}{V_2 \ (\text{Ao valve})}$$

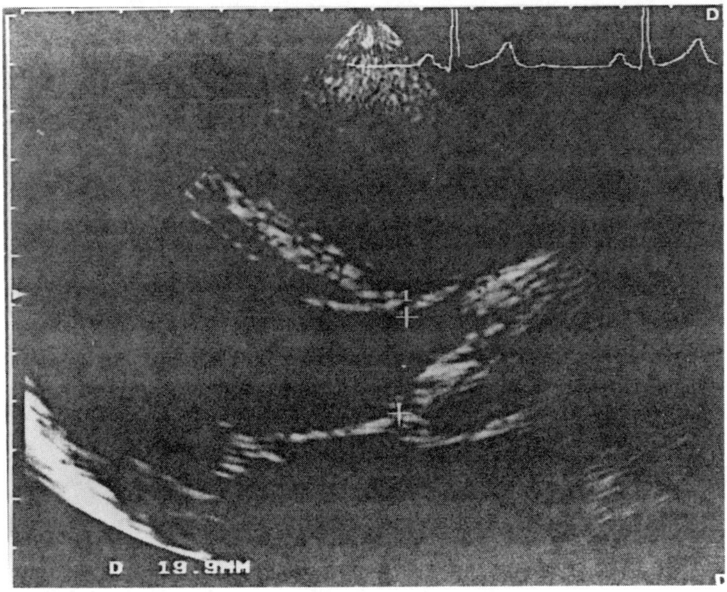

FIGURE 4. Measurement of the LVOT diameter (between markers +). This measurement was 1.99 cm. The LVOT area therefore equals

$$\pi r^2 = \left(\frac{d}{2}\right)^2 = \left(\frac{1.99}{2}\right)^2 = 3.10\ \text{cm}^2$$

LVOT area is determined by measuring the LVOT diameter (d) in midsystole where the anterior (right) aortic cusp joins the ventricular septum and where the posterior (noncoronary) aortic cusp joins the base of the anterior mitral valve leaflet as viewed on the parasternal long axis 2-D study (Figure 4). Then, the area is calculated as

$$A = \pi\, r^2 = 3.14\left(\frac{d}{2}\right)^2 = \text{cm}^2$$

Note that, since d is squared, small errors in the measurements of d can cause large errors in the calculation. Parenthetically, in adults, d will usually approximate 2 cm.

The LVOT flow velocity (V_1) is measured by pulsed wave Doppler (since accurate range-gated anatomic location is important), usually from the apical long axis view. In order to avoid the "prestenotic acceleration" which occurs close to the stenotic aortic valve, the Doppler sampling is started just below the valve and then backed down into the LVOT until a stable velocity is obtained (Figure 5). This is usually 1.0 to 1.5 cm below the valve. At this level the velocities across the entire LVOT are usually uniform.

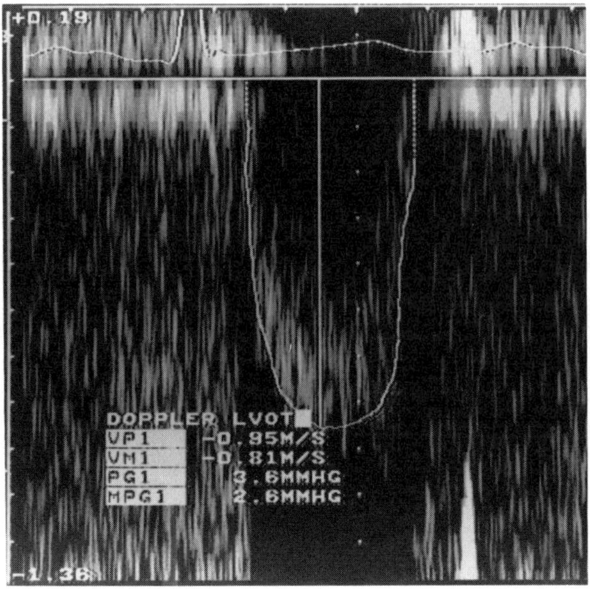

FIGURE 5. PW recording (apical long axis view) of LVOT systolic velocity (V_1). The recorded peak velocity is 0.95 m/s.

CW Doppler is utilized to obtain the maximum aortic flow velocity jet (Figure 6). This may be from apical, high right parasternal, or other views, wherever the *maximum* velocity is found ("it is impossible to record a velocity higher than maximum").

Utilizing values from the accompanying illustrations (Figures 4, 5, and 6), the aortic valve area may now be calculated:

$$\text{AVA} = \text{LVOT area} \times \frac{V_1}{V_2}$$

$$\text{AVA} = 3.10 \times \frac{0.95}{3.30} = 0.89 \text{ cm}^2$$

Correlation with cardiac catheterization is excellent[3] and where discrepancies occur it is usually with the larger valve areas (echo-Doppler usually finds smaller areas than do catheterization values). Recall, however, that the catheter-determined (Gorlin) values are not a perfect gold standard. The continuity equation may provide superior results especially if aortic valvular insufficiency is present or very high or very low COs are present.

In the continuity equation for AVA, as applied practically, note that V_1 (pulsed Doppler) is more likely to be overestimated (i.e., if the sample volume is placed in the area of prestenotic acceleration). This error would falsely *increase* the AVA. The V_2 is more likely to be underestimated since one may

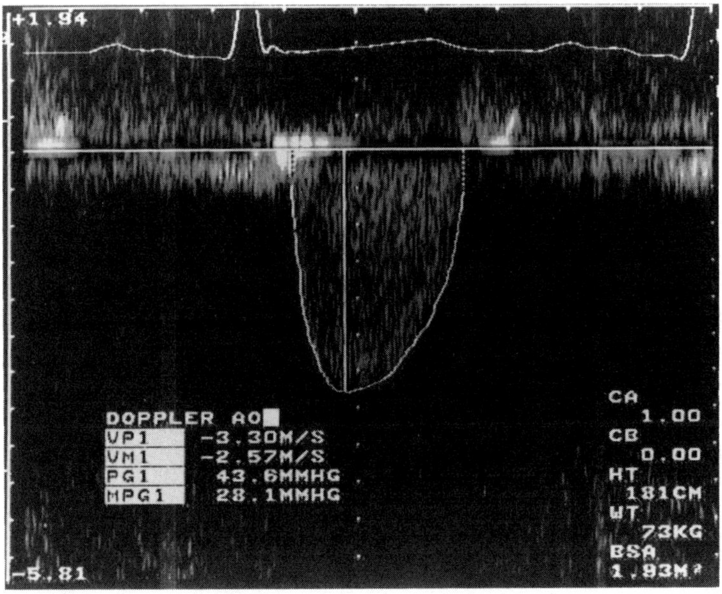

FIGURE 6. CW recording of the systolic flow velocity across a stenotic aortic valve (contains the velocities from the LVOT and aortic root, but the highest velocities as recorded will, of course, be from the stenotic aortic valve.) In this instance, a Vmax or peak velocity (V_2) of 3.30 m/s was recorded (normal is less than 1.9 m/s). This resulted in a peak gradient of 43.6 mmHg and a mean gradient of 28.1

not be parallel to flow and therefore may not obtain Vmax. This error would also tend to *increase* the AVA. Thus, the only likely way to falsely *decrease* the AVA would be to underestimate the diameter (or area) of the LVOT.

Values for AVA in aortic stenosis (AS) are expressed in different terms by different authors. We utilize the following:

Severity of AS (cm^2)

Mild	>1.2
Moderate	0.5–1.2
Severe	<0.5

Other authors[4] prefer the following terminology.

Severity of AS (cm^2)

absent	>2.2
insignificant	1.1–2.2
significant	<1.1

As noted above, in the continuity equation, the measurement of the diameter of the LVOT is a critical component. Where this measurement, for technical or other reasons, cannot be accurately determined, then one may utilize the V_1/V_2 ratios. Note this *ratio* is independent of CO since increases or decreases in output would affect V_1 and V_2 proportionately. In these instances the ratio is more accurate than gradient calculation. If no gradient is present, then this ratio should approximate unity. Where the V_1/V_2 ratio is less than 0.25, severe AS is usually present.[3] Note that these changes are just the reverse of pressure (P) changes in AS (V_1 is relatively low to V_2, whereas P_1 is relatively high to P_2).

C. AORTIC STENOSIS WITH INSUFFICIENCY

By increasing stroke output, aortic insufficiency (AI) will elevate the calculated AS gradient. Several methods are available for "correcting" these calculations. These include the following.

1. Subtracting Gradients

This may be accomplished by two methods. One is simply to subtract the LVOT gradient determined by pulsed Doppler (Figure 5) from the aortic valve gradient determined by CW Doppler (Figure 6). In this instance it is assumed that the LVOT gradient is that due to the AI. This would then correct for the AI influence on the AS gradient (i.e., changes in CO affect both gradients equally and therefore cancel out, similar to V_1/V_2 ratio).

Another method is to subtract the V_1 flow velocity from the V_2 flow velocity on a single CW aortic velocity study (Figure 7). The reasoning here is similar to that in the first method. Figure 8 presents these principles diagrammatically. In this illustration, V_1 is the velocity from the LVOT and can represent the contribution from AI, i.e., $4V^2 = 4(2)^2 = 16$ mmHg gradient from AI. This can be checked against the pulsed Doppler-determined LVOT gradient. The maximum "uncorrected" gradient (with a peak velocity of 5 m/s) would be $4V^2 = 4(5)^2 = 100$ mmHg. Therefore, the gradient corrected for AI is $100 - 16 = 84$ mmHg.

2. Flow Velocity Pattern Configuration and Time to Peak Relative to Time of Flow (t peak/tQ)

If the t peak/tQ exceeds 40 to 50% there is usually severe AS. In AS, an "early peak" implies the stenosis is mild and/or in the presence of a large gradient — there may be a significant contribution from AI — while a "late peak" indicates probably severe stenosis. A "very late peak" is characteristic of hypertrophic (dynamic) subaortic stenosis (Figure 9).

III. AORTIC INSUFFICIENCY (AI)

For several years the severity of AI lesions were semiquantitatively determined by pulsed Doppler "mapping" of the distribution of the AI jet back into

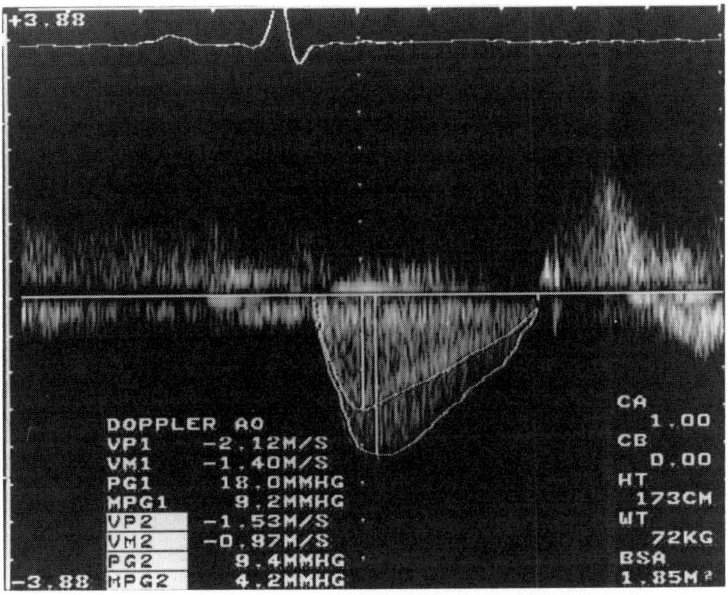

FIGURE 7. CW recording of systolic flow velocities across the LVOT and the aortic valve in a patient with mild AI and trivial AS. The peak recorded velocity is 2.12 m/s and the peak gradient is 18 mmHg. The contribution of the AI to the peak velocity is 1.53 m/s and to the gradient is 9.4 mmHg. Thus, the aortic systolic gradient "corrected" for AI would be only 18.0 – 9.4 = 8.6 mmHg (and therefore insignificant).

the LV cavity. This was time consuming and recent studies have shown the method also to be inaccurate. For example, by the pulsed method, the AI was thought to be severe if the jet could be detected at a distance far back into the LV cavity. Color Doppler studies have shown however that some of these jets were "pencil-like", extending a long distance, but were of small "volume". In other instances, color Doppler studies have revealed two or more jets and jets which may be oriented in relatively unusual directions (e.g., closely along the IV septum or closely along the anterior mitral leaflet) in which case the pulsed study may not interface with a significant area of the jet or indeed may miss the jet entirely. For these and other reasons most laboratories are using other means to quantitate the severity of AI.

Color Doppler mapping of the area of the AI jet (parasternal short-axis view) or the height of the AI jet (parasternal long-axis view) and relating this to the area and height of the LVOT, respectively, has been utilized[5] (Figure 10). In these determinations it is important to measure the jet just below the aortic valve, since the jet may "fan out" down in the cavity of the LV. These techniques are diagrammatically presented in Figure 11.

CW Doppler studies are also of value. Conventional CW of the AI jet displays the time of the jet on the "X" axis (m/s) and the velocity of the jet on

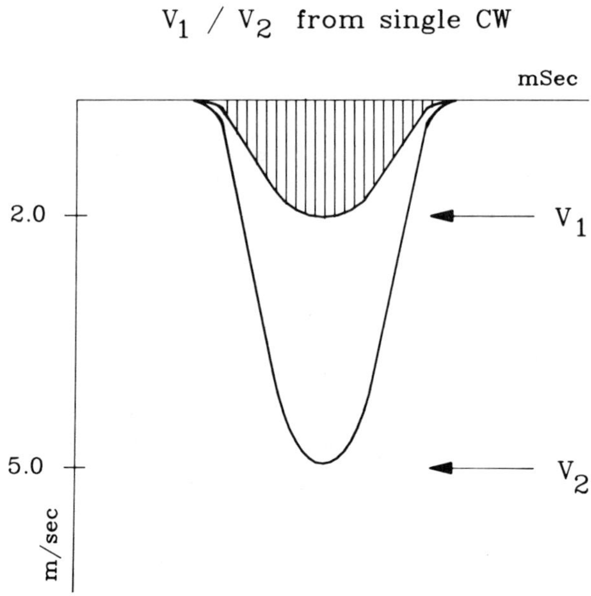

FIGURE 8. Diagrammatic representation of a CW-recorded systolic velocity flow profile from a patient with very severe AS complicated by AI. V2 is the Vmax recorded across the LVOT and aortic valve. V1 is the velocity profile from the LVOT. This velocity is presumed to be due to the AI. Thus, this gradient would be 4V2 = 4(2)2 = 16 mmHg. Therefore, the "corrected" aortic stenosis gradient would be 100 – 16 = 84 mmHg (still severe AS even when the gradient is "corrected" for the AI contribution).

the "Y" axis. The *intensity* (decibels) of the CW signal is displayed on the "Z" axis. In general, the more intense the AI signal, the more severe the AI (Figure 12). Note that the *rate* of change of the *gradient* (aortic root to LV) from early to late diastole (as aortic root pressure falls and the left ventricular pressure rises to the left ventricular end-diastolic pressure, LVEDP) will be slow if AI is mild and rapid if AI is severe (Figures 12 and 13). From the CW waveform the pressure half-time of the AI jet may be determined (also see Chapter 3). The more rapid the gradient change, the shorter will be the pressure half-time. Thus, *pressure half-times* can be utilized to judge the severity of the AI.

Severity of AI (Pressure Half-Time in m/s, AI)

Mild	>500
Moderate	200–500
Severe	<200

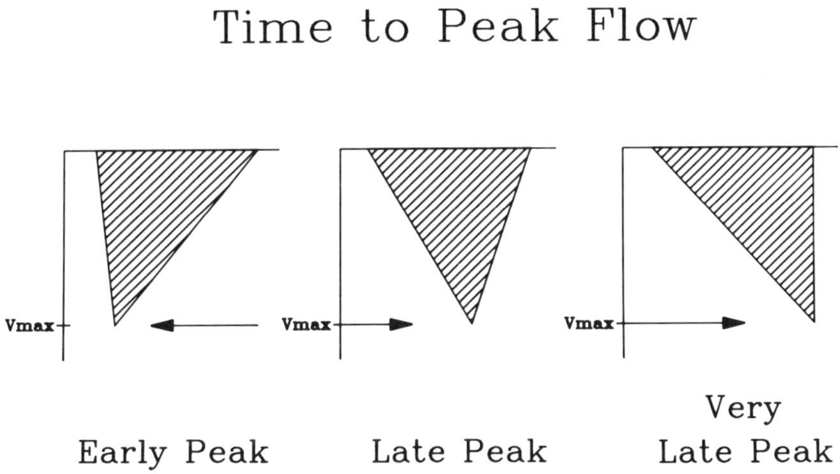

A

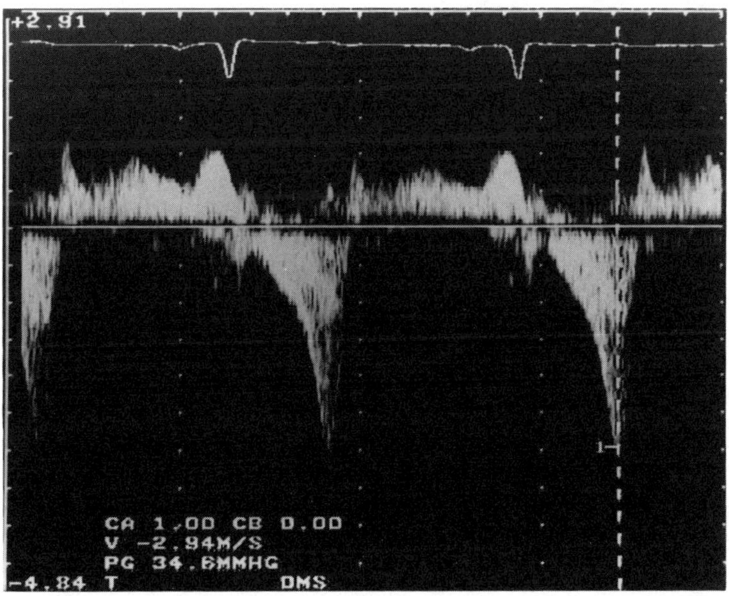

B

FIGURE 9. (A) Diagram of CW-recorded systolic flow velocity patterns across the LVOT and aortic valve in mild AS or AS where a high velocity has a large contribution from AI (left), severe AS (middle), and hypertrophic subaortic stenosis (right). (B) Actual CW recording from a patient with dynamic obstruction to the LVOT (hypertrophic subaortic stenosis). The peak gradient is 34.6 mmHg. Note particularly the crescendo development to peak late at the end of systole.

Aortic Insufficiency

Color Doppler

Severity of AI	Parasternal short axis $\frac{\text{area of jet}}{\text{area of LVOT}}$ %	Parasternal long axis $\frac{\text{height of jet}}{\text{height of LVOT}}$ %
Trivial	< 4	1 – 24
Mild	4 – 24	25 – 46
Moderate	25 – 59	47 – 64
Severe	> 60	> 65

FIGURE 10. Severity of AI as judged by the related height and area ratios (consult text and Figure 11).

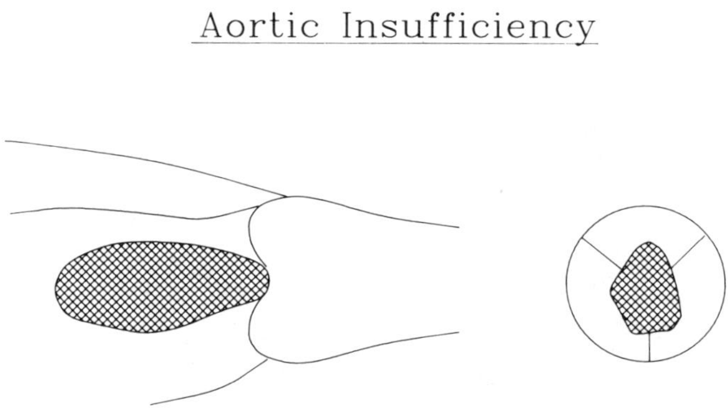

FIGURE 11. Diagrammatic illustration of color Doppler recording of AI in the parasternal long-axis view (PLAX) and the parasternal short-axis view (PSAX). In the PLAX the height of the AI jet is measured as 1.2 cm and the height of the LVOT is measured as 2.0 cm. Therefore, the height % is 1.2/2.0 = 60%, which is AI of moderate severity. In the PSAX the diameter of the LVOT is 2 cm and therefore the area = $\pi r^2 = 3.14\ (2/2)^2 = 3.14\ cm^2$. The area of the AI jet measured by planimetry is 1.9 cm^2. Therefore, the area % is 1.9/3.14 = 61%, again reflecting moderately severe AI.

In Figure 13, note the computer calculation of the pressure half-time (PHT) of the AI to be 74 ms, thus indicating severe AI.

Figure 14 presents a CW recording from a patient with moderate to severe AI. Note the rapid decline in gradient and the calculated relatively short pressure half-time (PHT) of 208 ms.

Aortic Insufficiency

CW Doppler

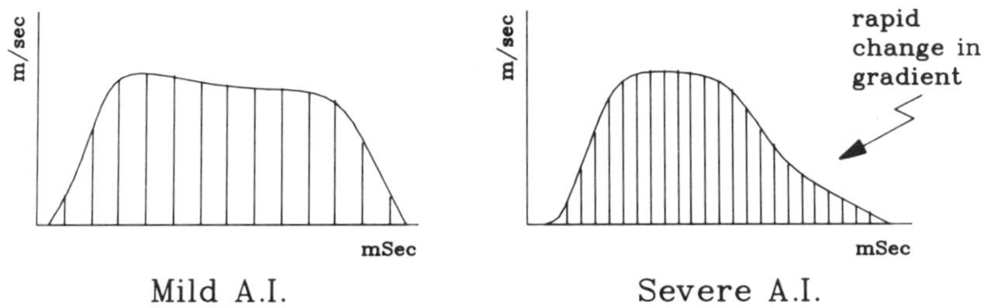

FIGURE 12. Diagrammatic illustration of mild AI compared to severe AI. Note the "intensity" of the signal (decibels or "brightness" of the jet velocity profile) is increased in severe AI. Also note the more rapid decline in aortic root to LV gradient in severe AI.

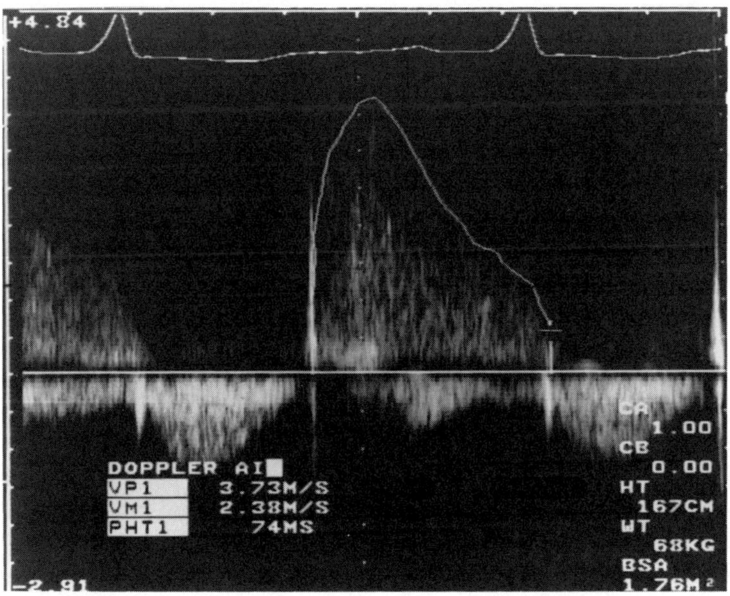

FIGURE 13. Actual CW recording of severe AI demonstrating the very rapid decline in the diastolic gradient.

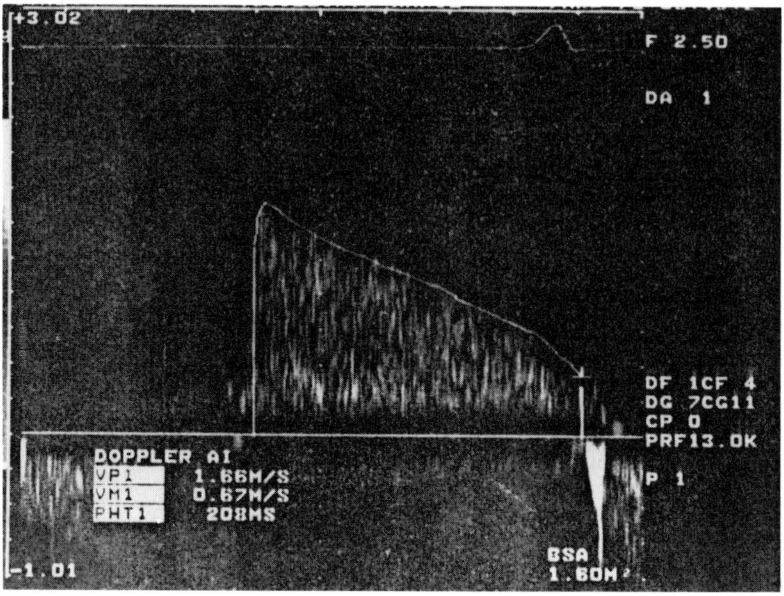

FIGURE 14. CW recording of moderate to severe AI. Note the high intensity of the signal. Also note the rapid decline of the gradient. Further, the Vmax of the AI was recorded at 1.66 m/s. Thus, $1.66/\sqrt{2} = 1.66/1.4 = 1.19$ m/s. The time taken for the Vmax to decline to 1.19 m/s (p1/2t) was 208 ms (calculation could be done by hand or, in the examples illustrated, the result was provided by the computer software program in the equipment). AI with a p1/2t of 208 ms would be moderate to severe.

The calculation of *AI regurgitant fractions* will be presented later (Chapter 10). Briefly,

$$\frac{SV_a - SV_p}{SV_a} \times 100 = \%\ \text{Regurgitant fraction}$$

where SV_a = aortic stroke volume and SV_p = pulmonic stroke volume.

IV. SUMMARY

Aortic Stenosis (AS)

The severity of aortic stenosis (AS) may be judged by the following:

A. *Max* instantaneous pressure *gradient* (CW) = $4V^2$.

B. *Mean gradient* (closer to catheter peak to peak), >50 mmHg is severe AS but gradient varies with CO.

Severity of AS (mean gradient, mmHg)

Mild	<20
Moderate	20–50
Severe	>50

C. *Continuity equation* for *aortic valve area* (AVA).

$$F = V \times A$$
$$V_1 \times \text{LVOT area} = V_2 \times \text{AVA}$$
$$\underset{(\text{cm}^2)}{\text{AVA}} = \underset{(\text{cm}^2)}{\text{LVOT area}} \times \frac{V_1\ (\text{LVOT})}{V_2\ (\text{AOR})}$$

Severity of AS (AVA, cm^2)

Mild	>1.2
Moderate	0.5–1.2
Severe	<0.5

D. *V_1/V_2 Ratios*

$\frac{V_1\ (\text{LVOT})}{V_2\ (\text{AOR})}$ = use this ratio when accurate area of LVOT cannot be obtained

$\frac{V_1}{V_2} < 0.25$ = severe AS (unlike) gradient, ratios do not change significantly with changes in CO).

nsufficiency (AI)

The severity of AI may be judged by

A. *Color Doppler*

Severity of AI	Area of jet to area of LVOT (SAX) (%)	Height of jet to height of LVOT (LAX) (%)
Trivial	<4	1–24
Mild	4–24	25–46
Moderate	25–59	47–64
Severe	>60	>65

B. *CW Doppler*

1. Intensity of AI signal.
2. Pressure half-times of AI jet in ms.

Mild >500
Moderate 200–500
Severe <200

C. *AI regurgitant fraction* (see Chapter 10)

SV_a = Aortic stroke volume.
SV_p = Pulmonic stroke volume.

$$\frac{SV_a - SV_p}{SV_a} \times 100 = \% \text{ Regurgitant fraction.}$$

REFERENCES

1. **Yoshida, K., et al.,** Color Doppler evaluation of valvular regurgitation in normal subjects, *Circulation,* 78, 840, 1988.
2. **Kostucki, W., Vandenbossche, J., Friart, A., and Englert, M.,** Pulsed Doppler regurgitant flow patterns of normal valves, *Am. J. Cardiol.,* 58, 309, 1986.
3. **Oh, J. K., et al.,** Prediction of the severity of aortic stenosis by Doppler aortic valve area determination, prospective Doppler-catheterization correlation in 100 patients, *J. Am. Coll. Cardiol.,* 1l, 1227, 1988.
4. **Warwick, J. M., et al.,** Clinical evaluation versus Doppler echocardiography in the quantitative assessment of valvular heart disease, *Circulation,* 78, 267, 1988.
5. **Perry, G. J., Helmcke, F., and Nanda, N. C., et al.,** Evaluation of aortic insufficiency by Doppler color flow mapping, *J. Am. Coll. Cardiol.,* 9, 952, 1987.

ADDITIONAL READING

Hatle, L., Angelsen, B. A., and Tromsdol, A., Non-invasive assessment of aortic stenosis by Doppler ultrasound, Br. Heart J., 43, 284, 1980.

Teirstein, P., Yeager, M., Yock, P., and Popp, R. L., Doppler echocardiograhic measurement of aortic valve area in aortic stenosis: a non-invasive application of the Gorlin formula, *J. Am. Coll. Cardiol.,* 8, 105, 1986.

Fan, P., Kapur, K. K., and Nanda, N. C., Color-guided Doppler echocardiographic assessment of aortic valve stenosis, *J. Am. Coll. Cardiol.,* 12, 441, 1988.

Beyer, R. W., Ramirez, M., Josephson, M. A., and Shah, P.M., Correlation of continuous wave Doppler assessment of chronic aortic regurgitation with hemodynamics and angiography, *Am. J. Cardiol.,* 60, 852, 1987.

Labovitz, A. J., et al., Quantitative evaluation of aortic insufficiency by continuous wave Doppler echocardiography, *J. Am. Coll. Cardiol.,* 8, 1341, 1986.

Assey, M. E., Usher, B. W., and Hendrix, G. H., Valvular heart disease: use of invasive and noninvasive techniques in clinical decision-making. I. Aortic valve disease, *Mod. Concepts Cardiovasc. Dis.,* 58, 55, 1989.

Currie, P. J., Hagler, D. J., and Seward, J. D., et al., Instantaneous pressure gradient: a simultaneous Doppler and dual catheter correlative study, *J. Am. Coll. Cardiol.,* 7, 800, 1986.

Chapter 6

MITRAL VALVE

I. INTRODUCTION

The normal mitral valve (MV) maximal diastolic flow velocity is usually less than 1.3 m/s. Although mitral stenosis (MS) is absent, "physiologic" mitral regurgitation (MR) may be detected by Doppler study in up to 40% of normal individuals.[1]

II. MITRAL STENOSIS (MS)

Methods to assist in gauging the severity of MS include planimetry of the orifice, determination of gradients (maximum, mean, and end diastolic), calculation of pressure half-time (P1/2t), and derivation of mitral valve area (MVA) by the P1/2t or by the continuity equation. Determination of pulmonary artery pressures (see Chapter 7) also assists in the evaluation of MS severity.

Using *planimetry* requires a 2-D echo scan of the mitral valve leaflets in diastole as studied in the parasternal short-axis view.[2] One determines the *minimum* orifice, then subjects this to planimetry (Figure 1). The normal adult MVA is 4 to 6 cm^2 (with variation in relation to body size). The MVA (cm^2) in MS may be graded as follows:[3]

Severity of MS (MVA in cm^2)

Mild	>1.8
Moderate	1.3–1.8
Severe	<1.3

Limitations to planimetry in assessing the severity of MS are present when there is extensive subvalvular disease (with thickened and shortened mitral chords) and/or with extensive annulus calcification (annular stenosis), either of which may produce diastolic obstruction to flow across the mitral apparatus.

Mitral diastolic flow velocities are easily determined in most instances. Utilizing the shortened Bernoulli equation ($4V^2$), the *maximum diastolic mitral gradient* may be calculated (Figure 2). Integration of the mitral diastolic flow display provides the *mean diastolic mitral gradient* (this calculation is usually provided in the computer software of modern equipment). Also from the velocity display, the *end-diastolic mitral gradient* may be calculated (Figure 2).

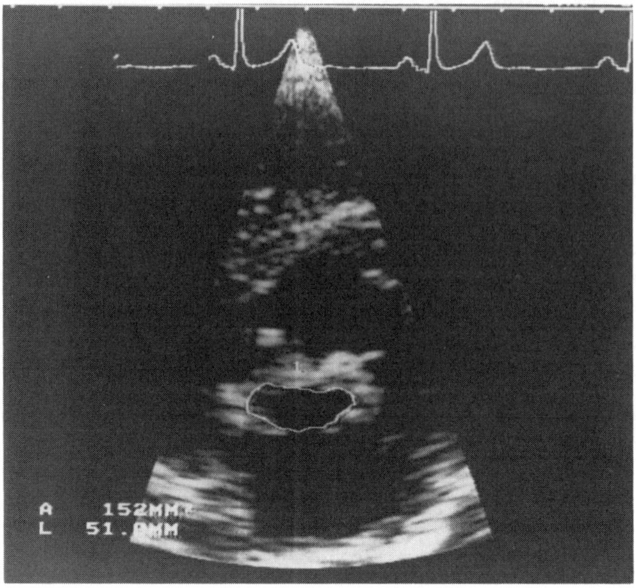

FIGURE 1. Mitral stenosis. Planimetry of the minimum mitral valve orifice detected on parasternal short-axis 2-D echo view. The orifice is electronically traced and computed by the equipment software to be 1.52 cm^2, mitral stenosis of moderate severity.

As noted in Chapter 3, the mitral diastolic P1/2t may be a better gauge of mitral stenosis than the gradients since the P1/2t is not influenced significantly by changes in heart rate and cycle length (lower end-diastolic and mean gradients with longer cycle lengths), cardiac output, or the presence of mitral regurgitation. P1/2t may not be accurate, however, in the presence of severe aortic regurgitation (as will be discussed later).

As indicated in Chapter 3, the mitral diastolic P1/2t may be derived from the diastolic velocity display. Two methods are in common use today. One method utilizes the following formula:

$$\frac{V\,max}{\sqrt{2}} = \frac{V\,max}{1.4} = \text{Velocity at P}\,1/2t$$

One then simply determines the time at which this velocity occurs and expresses this as the P1/2t (Figure 3).

Another method for determining the mitral diastolic P1/2t utilizes the following formula.[4]

$$0.29 \times \text{Deceleration time} = \text{P}\,1/2t$$

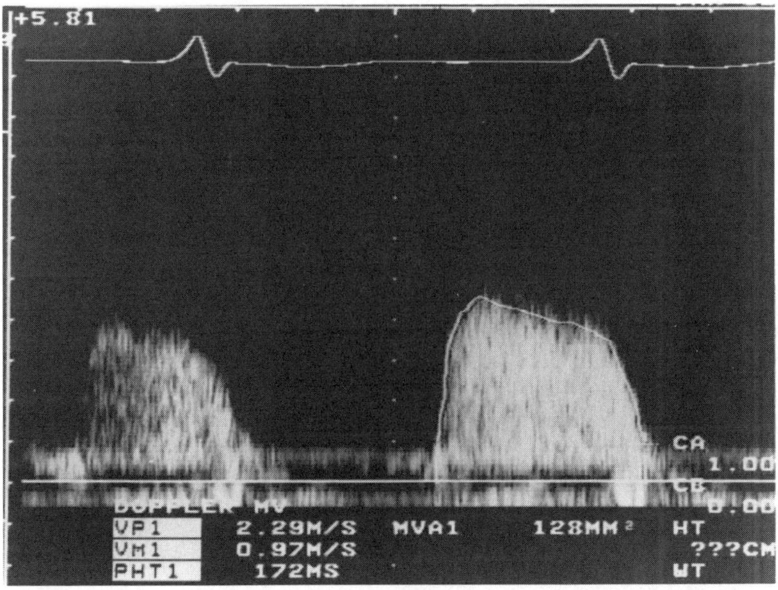

FIGURE 2. Mitral stenosis. Continuous wave Doppler recording of diastolic transmitral flow velocities. Vertical velocity markers at 0.5 m/s. A maximum diastolic velocity of 2.29 m/s was obtained. Using $4V^2 = 4(2.29)^2 = 21$ mmHg maximum diastolic gradient. An end-diastolic velocity of 1.8 m/s was recorded. Thus, $4(1.8)^2 = 13$ mmHg end-diastolic gradient.

Normal values for P1/2t are 20 to 60 m/s. In MS the values in m/s relative to the severity of the MS are

Severity of MS (P1/2t in m/s)

Mild	<180
Moderate	180–280
Severe	>280

It has been shown that a P1/2t of 220 equates to MS valve area orifice of approximately 1 cm^2.[5] Thus, the following formula for MVA may be utilized:

$$\text{MVA} = \frac{220}{\text{P}1/2\text{t}} = \text{cm}^2$$

and from the illustration in Figure 3:

$$\text{MVA} = \frac{220}{372} = 0.59\ \text{cm}^2$$

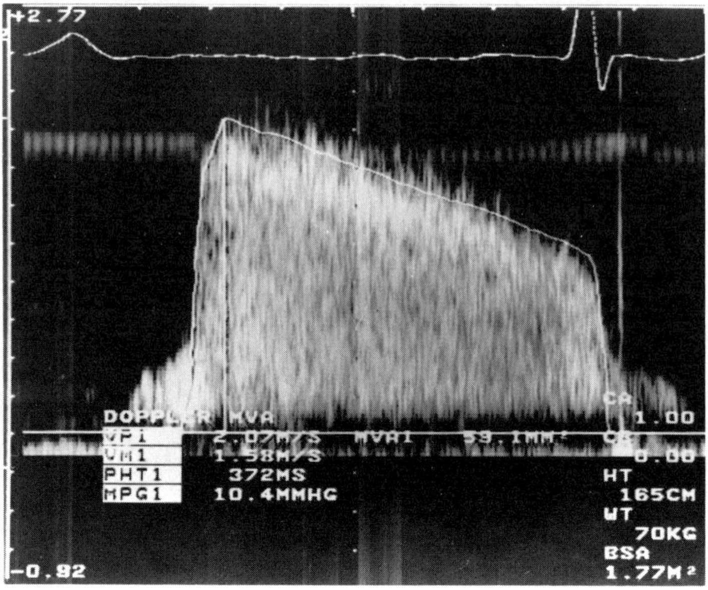

FIGURE 3. Mitral stenosis. Continuous wave Doppler recording of transmitral diastolic flow revealing a peak velocity of 2.07 m/s. Using the formula

$$\frac{\text{V max}}{\sqrt{2}} = \frac{2.07}{1.4} = 1.48 \text{ ms}$$

or the velocity at which P1/2t would occur. The time taken for the velocity to fall from 2.07 m/s to 1.48 m/s was 372 ms and this is then the P1/2t. Extrapolation of the deceleration curve from the start, down to the time baseline, provides the deceleration time, which in this instance is 1283 ms. Thus, using another method, i.e., 0.29 × deceleration time = 0.29 × 1283 = 372 ms = P1/2t. This would indicate severe MS.

A. DEPRESSURIZATION METHOD TO ASSESS THE SEVERITY OF MITRAL STENOSIS

The relationship between MVA and depressurization (deceleration) time is demonstrated in the formula[4]

$$\text{MVA}\left(\text{cm}^2\right) = \frac{751}{\text{depressurization time (ms)}}$$

According to the author[4] of this formula, it is simpler, more accurate, and easier to use (especially when atrial fibrillation is present) than the P1/2t method. In Figure 3 the deceleration time was 1283 ms, thus,

$$\text{MVA}\left(\text{cm}^2\right) = \frac{751}{1283} = 0.59 \text{ cm}^2$$

Using the above calculations, some authors have chosen to gauge the severity of MS as follows:[6]

Severity of MS (MVA in cm^2)

Absent	>2.2
Insignificant	1.5–2.2
Significant	<1.5

B. CONTINUITY EQUATION TO ASSESS THE SEVERITY OF MITRAL STENOSIS

The P1/2t determinations (and similar methods) produce a significant *overestimation* of the MVA in patients with associated moderate to severe aortic insufficiency (AI) and in such cases the continuity equation probably should be used to quantify the MVA noninvasively.[7] (See also the discussion of the continuity equation in Chapter 5.) It should be noted, however, that the continuity equation *underestimates* the MVA in patients with associated significant MR since MR produces augmentation of the Doppler measurement of the mitral flow time velocity integral (TVI, see Chapter 4). Therefore, in the absence of moderate to severe AI, the MVA calculated by the P1/2t is accurate and more practical to use than the continuity equation. With significant AI, however, the continuity equation is utilized as follows:

$$SV = TVI \times A$$

where SV is stroke volume (cc), TVI is the time velocity integral (cm), and A is area (cm^2). Recall that the TVI (Chapter 4) may be provided by equipment computer software integration of the flow profile or may be calculated as:

$$TVI = \text{mean } V \times ET$$

where mean V is the mean velocity of the flow profile and ET is the ejection time.

Relevant *areas* are the aortic annulus area (AAA) (measured on 2-D long axis, inner-inner, midsystole, base of cusps, for diameter, then πr^2) and the pulmonic annulus area (PAA) (measured on 2-D short axis, midsystole, base of cusps, for diameter, then πr^2). The "unknown" area, of course, is the MVA.

TVIs are angle corrected if the incident angle exceeds 20° and are indicated as TVIa = TVI aortic, TVIp = TVI pulmonic, and TVIm = TVI mitral.

Thus, in MS, stroke volume (SV) in accordance with the continuity equation (also see Chapter 5) are

$$SV_1 \text{ (stenotic)} = SV_2 \text{ (nonstenotic)}$$

$$SV = TVI \times A$$

Thus,

$$\text{MVA}\left(\text{cm}^2\right)\times\text{TV Im(cm)}=\text{AAA}\left(\text{cm}^2\right)\times\text{TVIa (cm)}$$

or

$$\text{MVA}=\frac{\text{AAA}\times\text{TVIa}}{\text{TVIm}}=\text{cm}^2$$

However, since significant AI enhances the TVIa (and would *overestimate* the MVA), then it is best to use the following formula:

$$\text{MVA}\times\text{TVIm}=\text{PAA}\times\text{TVIp}$$

or

$$\text{MVA}=\frac{\text{PAA}\times\text{TVIp}=\text{cm}^2}{\text{TV Im}}$$

An example of the application of the continuity equation in evaluating MS is shown in Figures 4A, B, and C. From these figures, the following values are derived: PAA = 3.8 cm^2, TVI_m = 1.23 cm, and TVI_p = 0.15 cm.

Therefore,

$$\text{MVA}=\frac{3.8\times0.15}{1.23}=0.46\ \text{cm}^2$$

which indicates severe MS.

It should be noted that in some patients the walls of the pulmonary artery (PA) may not be clearly identified and thus the diameter (d) of the PA cannot be accurately measured. In such instances one may just measure the excursion of the posterior (left) pulmonic valve cusp (usually easily visualized) and assume this is the radius (r) of the PA.[8]

To summarize, in the *quantitation of MS,* the following guidelines may be utilized.

1. If there is no MR and no AI, then use the P1/2t method since it is simple and accurate.
2. If there is moderate to advanced MR, use the P1/2t method since the continuity equation (TVIm portion) would not be accurate.
3. If there is moderate to advanced AI, then use the continuity equation since the P1/2t method would not be accurate. In the continuity equation, in this instance, use the TVIp and not the TVIa.

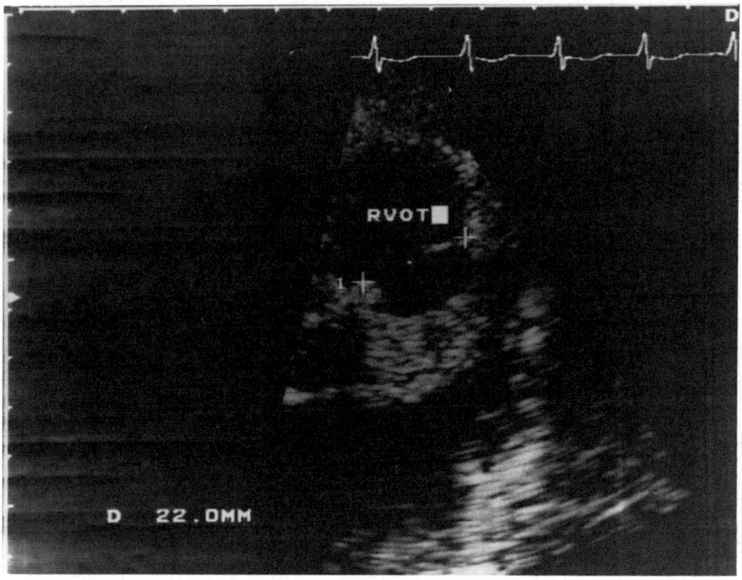

A

FIGURE 4. (A) 2-D parasternal short-axis view at the level of aortic valve and pulmonary artery (PA). The PA is measured between the markers (+) with a diameter of 22 mm = 2.2 cm. Thus, PAA = $\pi r^2 = 3.14\ (2.2/2)^2 = 3.8\ cm^2$. (B) Continuous wave Doppler recording of diastolic transmitral flow. Time-line markers are at 0.1 s. The diastolic flow occurs over a period of 0.77 s. The mean velocity of flow is 1.6 m/s. Thus, the TVIm = $160 \times 0.77 = 123.2$ cm. (C) Pulsed wave Doppler recording of systolic flow in the PA just above the pulmonic valve. The time markers are at 0.1 s. The ET is 0.33 s. The mean velocity is 0.45 m/s. Therefore, the TVIp = $0.45 \times 0.33 = 0.15$ cm.

4. If there is concomitant moderate to advanced MR and AI then one may utilize both the P1/2t method and the continuity equation (TVIp portion) and take the average of the two (although this technique requires clinical validation).

III. MITRAL REGURGITATION (MR)

Theoretic and practical limitations notwithstanding, the severity of MR may be assessed by the following means.

1. *Color Doppler*-determined MR jet area (MRJA) in relation to the left atrial area (LAA), the areas being planimetered or visually estimated.[9] This represents the "distribution" or "dispersal" of the blood cells in the MR jet. The MRJA is determined in the 2-D echo plane in which the jet area is the largest. The relationship then is as follows:

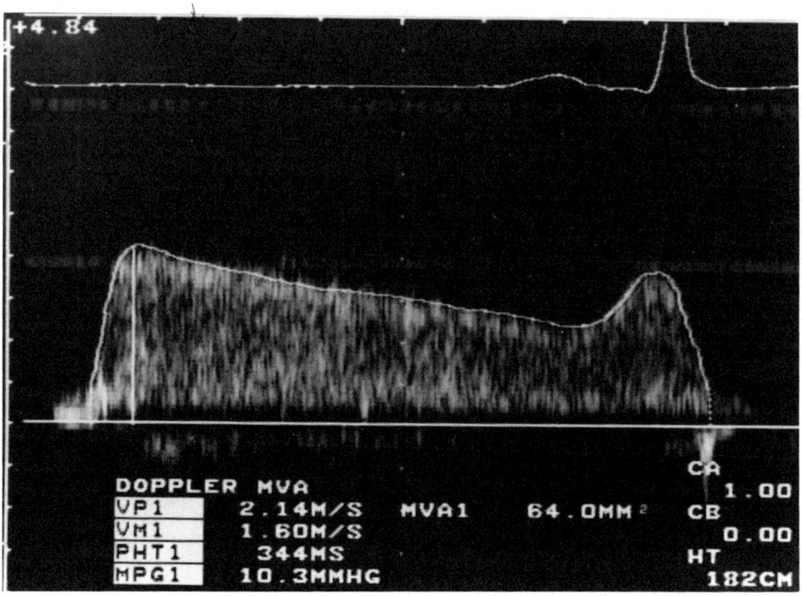

FIGURE 4B.

Severity of MR	MRJA/LAA %
Mild	<20
Moderate	20–40
Severe	>40

Figure 5 represents an example of severe MR.

2. *Direction* of the MR jet on color Doppler. "Physiologic" jets are usually small in volume and are directed posteriorly and medially into the left atrium[10] (Figure 6).
3. *Duration* of the MR. This time interval is on the "X" axis and can be determined by appropriate wave-form measurement or on an M-mode flow (M-Q) study. MR of less than 100 m/s and occurring very early in systole is usually "physiologic" (likely representing MV "seating" at closure in most). Jets of long duration indicate significant MR (Figures 6 and 7).
4. *Velocity* of the MR jet. The velocity of the jet is represented on the "Y" axis in m/s. This represents how fast the blood cells are moving. With MR of any significance the MR jet velocity usually exceeds 1.5 m/s. Jets of "physiologic" MR usually have velocities under 1.5 m/s (this generally measured by pulsed Doppler, since continuous wave Doppler (CW) may record these jets at over 1.5 m/s). Figure 7 illustrates an MR jet of high velocity. It should be noted that high-velocity jets may be recorded in some cases where the MR is of minimal severity. In such cases

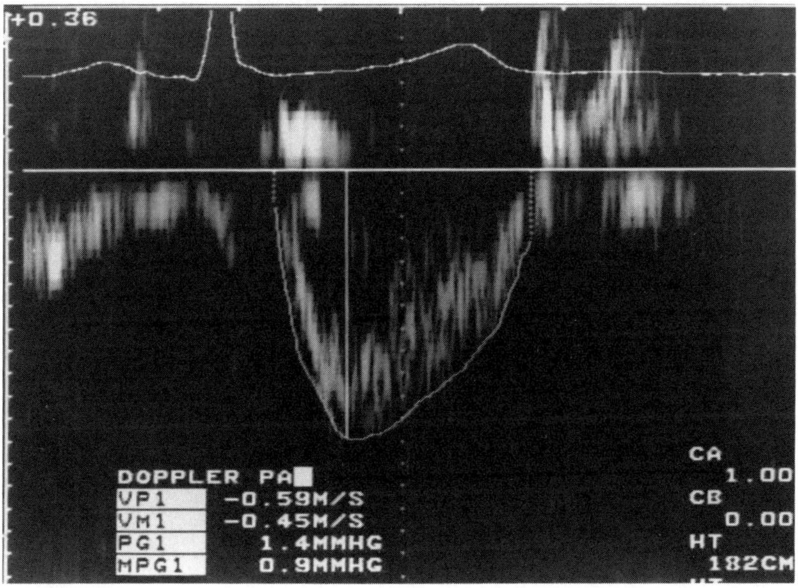

FIGURE 4C.

however the duration of the jet is usually short, the MRJA/LAA is small, and/or the intensity of the signal of the MR jet is low. Also, in some instances of "wide-open" MR, the recorded velocities may be relatively low; however, other parameters would clearly detect these very severe MRs (e.g., "volume" of regurgitant jet, increase in mitral diastolic flow, etc.). Of interest, prosthetic device paravalvular MR jets of relatively *small* volume may present velocities exceeding 5 m/s, therefore, with LV to LA gradientes exceeding 100 mmHg. In such cases, subtracting this gradient from the arm cuff recorded arterial systolic BP would yield the LA pressure.

5. *Intensity* of the MR signal. This is presented on the "Z" axis in decibels and is related to the number of blood cells in the MR jet. An intense jet (Figure 7) is more likely not to be of physiologic origin.
6. *Increase in diastolic flow* across the MV (i.e., flow velocities exceeding 1.3 m/s) are anticipated with significant MR. This increased flow velocity is distinguished from that due to MS in that with MR, although the Vmax in diastole may be high, there is a rapid deceleration (vs. prolonged in MS).
7. *Left atrial (LA) and left ventricular (LV) cavitary size* increases with increased LV contractility are anticipated in significant MR, however, these are influenced by factors such as the presence of acute vs. chronic MR, the presence or absence of atrial fibrillation (likely to be associated with more LA enlargement), and other factors.

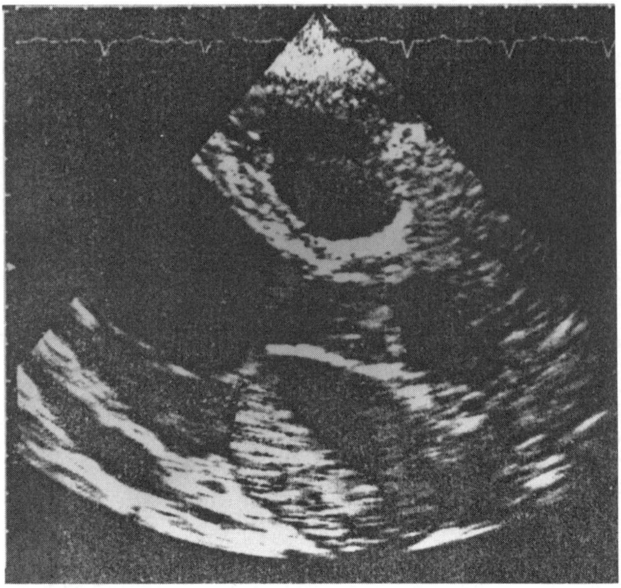

A

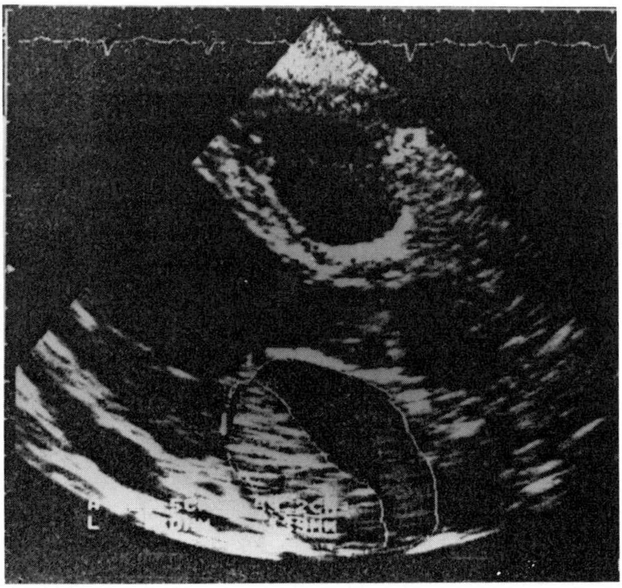

B

FIGURE 5. Severe MR. Black and white image derived from color flow study during systole, parasternal long-axis view, in a patient with severe MR. By visual estimation alone the MRJA/LAA approaches 50%. (A) Initial image. (B) Image subjected to planimetry.

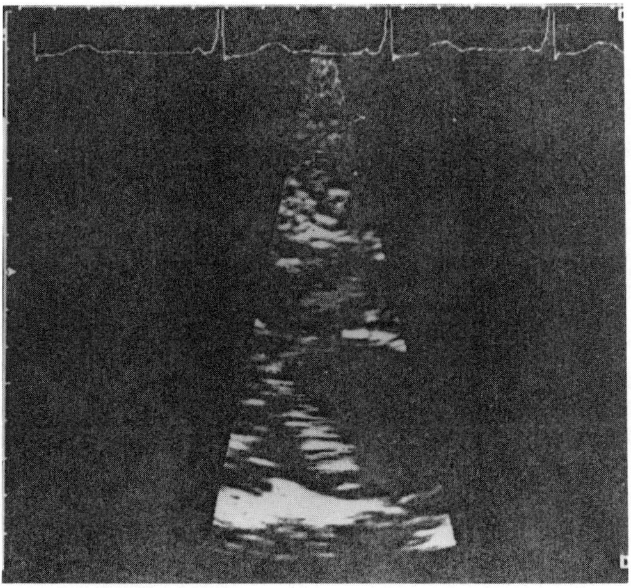

FIGURE 6. Direction of MR jet. Black and white image derived from color flow study, parasternal long axis, primarily of MV and left atrium. This is an MR jet of "small volume", directed posteriorly (also medially on the parasternal short-axis view) and relatively short duration (approximately 150 m/s).

8. On color Doppler, those jets displaying *"turbulence" (variance)* are likely to be pathologic.
9. *MR regurgitant fractions* (discussed later in Chapter 10). Briefly,

$$RF = \frac{LVSV - ASV}{LVSV} \times 100 = \%\ \text{regurgitant fraction}$$

ASV = aortic stroke volume (Doppler) and LVSV = left ventricular stroke volume (2-D-Simpson or M-Teicholz).

IV. SUMMARY

Mitral Stenosis (MS)

A. Pressure half-times (P1/2t)

$$1.\ \frac{Vmax}{\sqrt{2}} = \frac{V\,max}{1.4} = \text{Velocity at P1 / 2t}$$

thus measure the time at which this velocity occurs = P1/2t

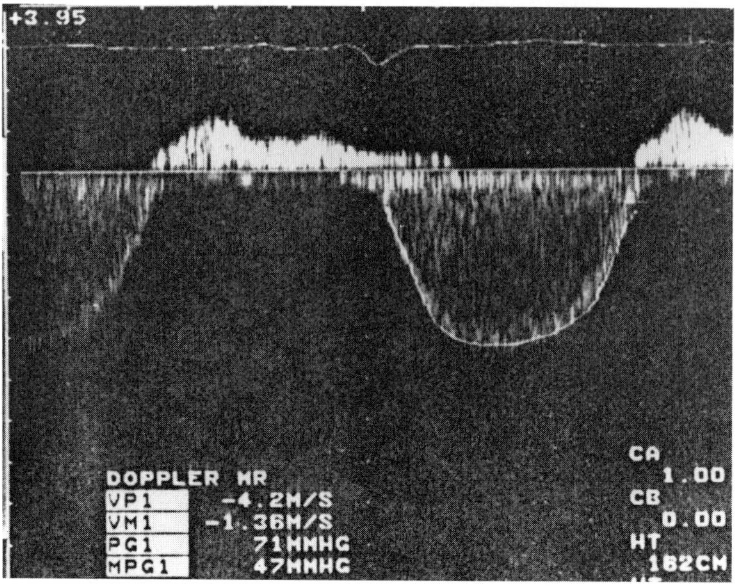

FIGURE 7. Severe MR. Continuous wave Doppler recording across the MV during systole revealing MR of fairly high intensity ("Z" axis, decibels), long duration (340 m/s) and high velocity (Vmax = 4.2 m/s).

2. $0.29 \times \text{Deceleration time} = \text{P1} / 2\text{t}$

B. Mitral valve area (MVA) calculated from the P1/2t:

$$\text{MVA} = \frac{220}{\text{P1} / 2\text{t}} = \text{cm}^2$$

C. Mitral valve area (MVA) calculated from the deceleration (depressurization) time:

$$\text{MVA} = \frac{751}{\text{depressurization time (ms)}} = \text{cm}^2$$

D. Continuity equation for MVA:

$$\text{SV}_1 \text{ (stenotic)} = \text{SV}_2 \text{(non - stenotic)}$$
$$\text{SV} = \text{TVI} \times \text{A}$$

and using the mitral and the pulmonary artery measurements:

$$MVA \times TVI_m = PAA \times TVI_p$$

or

$$MVA = \frac{PAA \times / TVI_p}{TVIm} = cm^2$$

E. Severity of MS (MVA, cm^2)

Mild	>1.8
Moderate	1.3–1.8
Severe	<1.3

Mitral Regurgitation (MR)

The severity of MR may be judged by the following:

1. MR color map

Severity of MR	MRJA/LAA (%)
Mild	<20
Moderate	20–40
Severe	>40

2. Direction of MR jet
Physiologic is usually posteriorly and medially into the LA.
3. Duration of MR jet
Less than 100 m/s is usually "physiologic".
4. Velocity of MR jet
"Physiologic" MR jet velocities are usually under 1.5 m/s (pulsed Doppler).
5. Intensity of the MR signal
"Z" axis in decibels.
6. Increase in Mitral Diastolic Flow
Flow exceeding 1.3 m/s. High peak but rapid deceleration (vs. MS).
7. LA and LV sizes
Acute vs. chronic MR, atrial fibrillation, and LV contractility.
8. "Turbulence" (variance) on color Doppler when present, more likely to be significant MR.
9. MR regurgitant fraction (RF) (see Chapter 10)

ASV = aortic stroke volume (Doppler) and LVSV = left ventricular stroke volume (2-D-Simpson or M-Teicholz).

REFERENCES

1. **Kostucki, W., Vandenbossche, J., Friart, A., and Englert, M.,** Pulsed Doppler regurgitant flow patterns of normal valves, *Am. J. Cardiol.,* 58, 309, 1986.
2. **Henry, W. L. and Griffith, J. M., et al.,** Measurement of mitral orifice area in patient with mitral valve disease by realtime, two-dimensional echocardiography, *Circulation,* 51, 827, 1975.
3. **Hagan, A. D. and DeMaria, A. N.,** *Clinical Applications of Two-Dimensional Echocardiography and Cardiac Doppler,* Little, Brown, Boston 1989.
4. **Pearlman, J. D. and Gibson, R.,** Doppler measurement of left atrial depressurization and mitral valve area in patients with suspected mitral stenosis: validation of a new method, *Am. Heart J.,* 113, 868, 1987.
5. **Hatle, L., Angelsen, B., and Tromsdal, A.,** Non-invasive assessment of atrioventricular pressure half-time by Doppler ultrasound, *Circulation,* 60, 1096, 1979.
6. **Warwick, J. M., et al.,** Clinical evaluation versus Doppler echocardiography in the quantitative assessment of valvular heart disease, *Circulation,* 78, 267, 1988.
7. **Nakatani, S., et al.,** Value and limitations of Doppler echocardiography in the quantification of stenotic mitral valve area: comparison of the pressure half-time and the continuity equation methods, *Circulation,* 77, 78, 1988.
8. **Giroud, J., Pickoff, A. S., and Ferrer, P. L.,** Pulsed Doppler echocardiographic quantification of left-to-right shunts in children with isolated ventricular septal defect. in *Cardiac Doppler Diagnosis,* Spencer, M. P., Ed., Martinius Nijhoff, The Hague, 227,
9. **Helmcke, F. and Nanda, N. C., et al.,** Color Doppler assessment of mitral regurgitation with orthogonal planes, *Circulation,* 75, 175, 1987.
10. **Yoshida, K., et al.,** Color Doppler evaluation of valvular regurgitation in normal subjects, *Circulation,* 78, 840, 1988.

ADDITIONAL READING

Libanoff, A. J. and Robard, S., Atrioventricular pressure half-time measure of mitral valve orifice area, *Circulation,* 38, 144, 1968.

Halbe, D., Bryg, R. J., and Labovitz, A. J., A simplified method for calculating mitral valve area using Doppler echocardiography, Am. Heart J., 116, 877, 1988.

Spain, M. G., et al., Quantitative assessment of mitral regurgitation by Doppler color flow imaging: angiographic and hemodynamic correlations, *J. Am. Coll. Ccardiol.,* 13, 585, 1989.

Chapter 7

PULMONIC VALVE, TRICUSPID VALVE, AND PRESSURES IN THE RIGHT ATRIUM, RIGHT VENTRICLE, AND PULMONARY ARTERY

I. PULMONIC VALVE (PV)

A. PULMONIC VALVULAR STENOSIS (PS)

The hemodynamic measurement of greatest value in determining the severity of PS is the gradient across this valve. The maximum systolic velocity (Vmax) across the PV (normally less than 0.9 m/s) is usually attained with ease by recording [best with continuous wave Doppler (CW)] the velocity profile across the valve as imaged from the parasternal short-axis view at the level of the PV and pulmonary artery. Applying the formula $4V^2$, one may determine the peak gradient. The severity of PS can then be judged as

Severity of PS (gradient, mmHg)

Mild	<40
Moderate	40–100
Severe	>100

Figure 1 illustrates PS of moderate severity.

B. PULMONIC VALVULAR INSUFFICIENCY (PI)

"Physiologic" PI may be recorded on Doppler studies in up to 92% of normal patients.[1] "Pathologic" PI is usually due to pulmonary hypertension. The severity of the PI may be judged on color Doppler by the distance the PI jet extends below the PV into the RV outflow tract, the "area" or "volume" of the jet, the presence of aliasing (red to blue) indicating a high velocity, the presence of turbulence or variance (mosaic) in the jet, and the duration of the PI. Although usually not done for clinical purposes, by CW one may measure the peak and mean velocities of the jet and the pressure half-time (P1/2t). As with AI (see Chapter 5) the deceleration rate of the PI spectral display relates directly to the severity of the PI or, stated differently, the more gradual the decline, the milder the PI. Figure 2 illustrates an example of PI of mild severity.

II. TRICUSPID VALVE (TV)

A. TRICUSPID VALVULAR STENOSIS (TS)

Although this is a rare disorder, TS may be evaluated by Doppler techniques similar to those utilized in the evaluation of mitral stenosis (MS). After record-

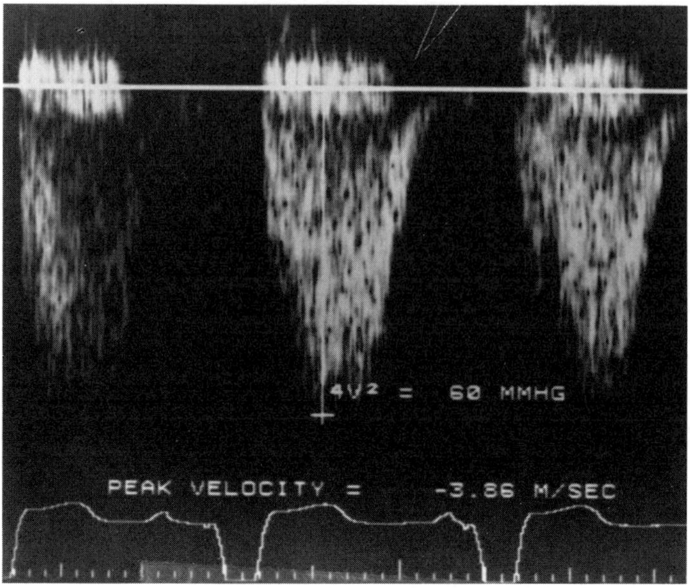

FIGURE 1. CW recording (parasternal short axis) across the PV in a patient with moderately severe PS. A peak velocity of 3.86 m/s was recorded (normal is <0.9 m/s). Using $4V^2$ produced a gradient of 60 mmHg.

ing the highest velocity (Vmax) of the TS jet (usually parasternal right ventricle (RV) inflow, parasternal short axis of the TV or apical 4-chamber views), then one may calculate the peak gradient ($4V^2$), the P1/2t, and the TV area (TVA) where:

$$TVA = \frac{220}{P1/2} = cm^2$$

The normal TVA is 5 to 8 cm^2.

B. TRICUSPID VALVULAR REGURGITATION (TR)

"Physiologic" TR may be recorded on Doppler studies in up to 95% of normal patients.[2] Indeed, it is frequently difficult to decide which instances of TR are "physiologic" and which are "pathologic", the latter usually associated with pulmonary hypertension. The severity of TR may be gauged by techniques similar to those used to evaluate mitral regurgitation (see Chapter 6) which include:

1. Color Doppler map of TR jet area in relationship to the RA area[3] (generally >35% is severe).

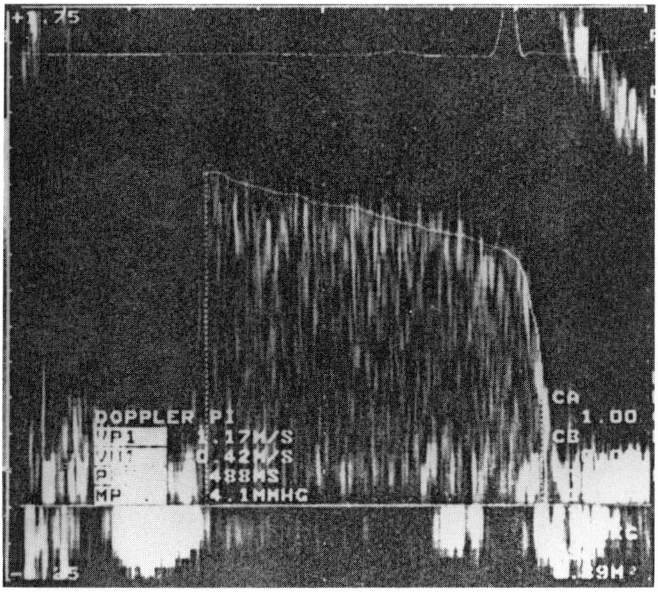

FIGURE 2. CW recording across the PV during diastole, revealing mild PI (note the gradual deceleration). The early velocity is 1.17 m/s and the end-diastolic velocity is 0.88 m/s. The end-diastolic gradient between the PA and the RV = $4V^2 = 4(0.88)^2 = 3.1$ mmHg. Assuming an RVEDP of 5 mmHg, then $3.1 + 5 = 8.1$ mmHg as the PA diastolic pressure. This pressure, of course, approximates the pulmonary capillary wedge pressure and the LVEDP.

2. Duration of the TR jet (e.g., exceeding 100 ms before being considered significant).
3. Velocity of the TR jet and evidence of aliasing on the color study. Recall that the TR *velocity* (determined by pulsed or CW Doppler) in "physiologic" TR may be just as high as that due to severe TR; however, the *intensity* of the signal would be significantly greater in severe TR (item #5). The velocity of the TR jet relates to the pressure gradient between the RV and right atrium (RA) rather than to the volume of the TR jet. An increased velocity, however, does help to distinguish TR from the lower velocities produced by "valve seating" (usually of low velocity and short duration).
4. Evidence of turbulent or variant flow (mosaic) in the TR jet on color Doppler usually indicates that the TR is not "physiologic"; however, when there is a large regurgitant orifice the retrograde flow from the RV to RA is usually laminar (since the pressure *differential* between RV and RA is small and therefore little turbulence is created). This latter observation is usually best appreciated on pulsed Doppler study.

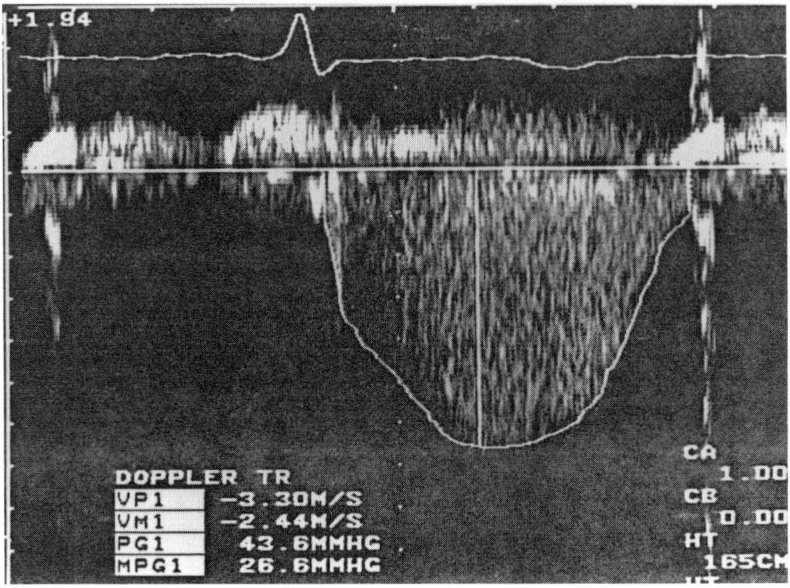

FIGURE 3. CW recording of TR of *moderate* severity. Note the long duration of the jet (460 m/s), the high velocity of the jet (Vmax = 3.3 m/s), and the high intensity of the TR signal, however, with a velocity profile not indicating this TR to be in the severe or advanced category.

5. Intensity of the TR signal on CW study (decibels on Z axis).
6. TR velocity profile (pulsed or CW). The more severe the TR the greater the tendency for a rapid upstroke and a rapid deceleration (due to the rapid and large increase in RA pressure with significant TR).
7. Increase in diastolic flow velocity across the TV (e.g., flow velocities exceeding the upper limit of normal Vmax of 0.8 m/s).
8. Evidence of flow reversal (pulsed or color Doppler) in the IVC and hepatic veins.
9. RA and RV cavity size enlargement, RV hyperdynamic motion and abnormal septal motion, secondary to RV volume overload.
10. Regurgitant fraction (see Chapter 10).

Figure 3 illustrates an example of TR of moderate severity.

III. PRESSURES IN THE RIGHT ATRIUM, RIGHT VENTRICLE, AND PULMONARY ARTERY

A. RIGHT ATRIAL PRESSURE (RAP)

The right atrial pressure (RAP) may be estimated by observation of the jugular venous pulse or by 2D-Doppler means. The RAP may be estimated at the Doppler exam by two methods. One method relates to the severity of any TR usually determined by color flow mapping. Thus, one could estimate RAP as follows:

Trivial TR	5 mmHg RAP
Mild TR	10 mmHg RAP
Moderate TR	15 mmHg RAP
Severe TR	20 mmHg RAP

A more reliable method for estimating the RAP deals with determining the size ("congested" or not) of the inferior vena cava (IVC) and whether or not there is a decrease in size of the IVC during inspiration (or a "sniff"). The IVC values are as follows (determined from the 2-D imaging study, subxyphoid view, measured within 2 cm of the IVC entrance to the RA):

Nondilated	<1.5 cm
Borderline	1.5–2.0 cm
Dilated	>2.0 cm
Decrease with deep inspiration	
Normal	>50%
Abnormal	<50%

Thus, relative to the IVC observations the RAP can be estimated as follows:

Nondilated	5 mmHg RAP
Borderline	5–10 mmHg RAP
Dilated with normal inspiratory variation	10–15 mmHg RAP
Dilated with abnormal inspiratory variation	15–20 mmHg RAP

B. RIGHT VENTRICULAR PRESSURE (RVP)

The right ventricular systolic pressure (RVP) may be estimated (see Chapter 2) by the formula:

$$G + RAP = RVP$$

where G is the TR determined maximum gradient ($4V^2$) across the TV during systole. Figures 4 and 5 illustrate this calculation.

C. PULMONARY ARTERY PRESSURE (PAP)

In the absence of PS, the RV systolic pressure (above) will be equal to the *systolic PAP* (Figure 4).

The following formula may be utilized to calculate the *mean PAP* (MPAP).[4]

$$MPAP = 80 - 1/2AT = mmHg$$

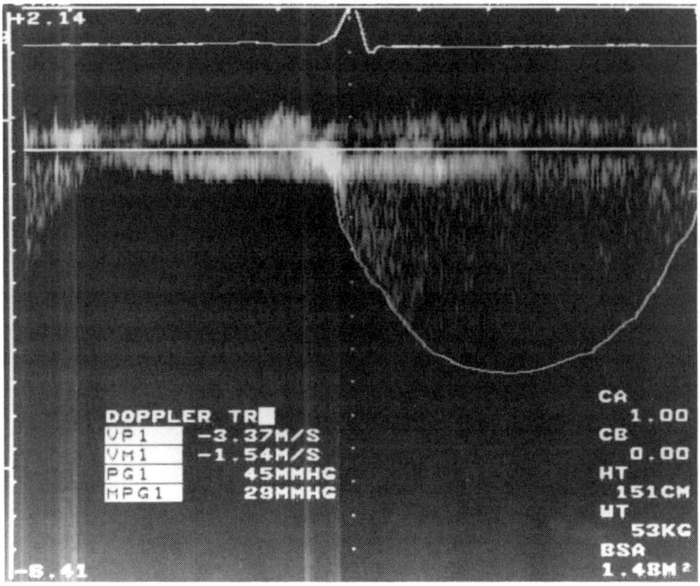

FIGURE 4. CW recording of TR to be used in calculation of pulmonary artery pressure. The Vmax of the TR = 3.37 m/s. Utilizing $4V^2 = 4(3.37)^2 = 45$ mmHg systolic gradient across the TV. The IVC in this patient measured 1.87 cm (see Figure 5), allowing an estimation of RAP of 10 mmHg. Thus, G + RAP = RVP or 45 + 10 = 55 mmHg right ventricular systolic pressure and, in the absence of PS, this is also the systolic PAP.

where AT is the acceleration time (in ms) of the PA flow velocity curve taken from the parasternal short-axis view at the level of the PV. This may be derived from the CW study or, more commonly, from the pulsed Doppler study with the sample volume placed in the PA just distal to the PV cusps or, perhaps better placed, in the RV outflow tract just below the PV. (Figure 6 illustrates this calculation). Parenthetically, a PA acceleration time of over 120 ms is usually normal, one less than 100 ms usually indicates pulmonary hypertension, and one less than 75 ms correlates with severe pulmonary hypertension.

Another method for calculating mean PAP is similar to the above as:[5]

$$\text{MPAP} = 90 - (0.62 \times \text{AT}) = \text{mmHg}$$

Diastolic PAP (DPAP) may be established as follows (see Chapter 2 for details):

$$\text{DPAP} - \text{RVDP} = \text{G}$$

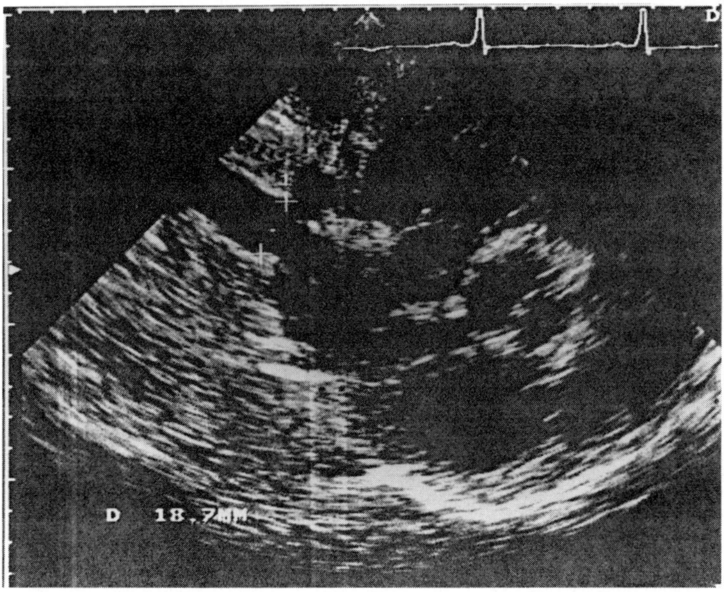

FIGURE 5. 2-D subxyphoid view of IVC entering the RA. The IVC measures 1.87 cm. This is borderline dilated, thus allowing an estimate of the RAP of 10 mmHg (also see Figure 4).

where RVDP is the RV diastolic pressure and G is the diastolic (late rather than early or peak) gradient between the PA and the RV. Therefore:

$$DPAP = G + RVDP$$

and RVDP is judged equivalent to RAP (estimated by techniques described in Chapter 2). In Figure 2 the jet is recorded at 0.88 m/s. Thus, $4V^2 = 4(0.88)^2 =$ 3 mmHg. Assume an RVDP of 5.0 mmHg, then 3 + 5 = 8 mmHg, a normal PA diastolic pressure.

IV. SUMMARY

Pulmonic stenosis (PS)

Determine Vmax, then gradient = $4V^2$ = mmHg.

Severity of PS (gradient, mmHg)

Mild	<40
Moderate	40–100
Severe	>100

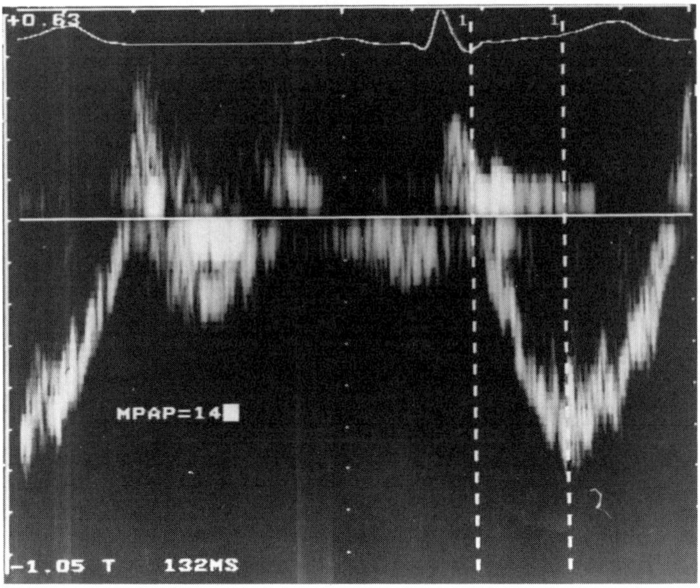

FIGURE 6. Pulsed wave recording of PA systolic flow profile with sample volume placed in the PA just distal to the pulmonic valve. Note an acceleration time (AT) of 132 ms. Utilizing the formula noted, the MPAP = 80 – 1/2 AT = 80 – 66 = 14 mmHg, a normal pressure.

Pulmonic insufficiency (PI)

Severity of PI may be judged by:

1. Distance jet extends from PV into RV outflow tract
2. The "area" or "volume" of the jet
3. High jet velocity, aliasing
4. Jet turbulence, mosaic
5. Duration of PI jet

Tricuspid stenosis (TS)

$$\text{TVA} = \frac{220}{\text{P1} / 2\text{t}} = \text{cm}^2$$

Normal TVA = 5 to 8 cm^2.

Tricuspid regurgitation (TR)

The severity of TR may be judged by:

1. Color Doppler jet area in relationship to the RA (generally >35% is severe).
2. Duration of TR jet (less than 100 ms probably not significant).
3. Velocity of TR jet and evidence of aliasing on color Doppler (exceptions noted in text).
4. Turbulent or variant (mosaic) flow in the TR jet on color Doppler (exceptions noted in text).
5. Intensity of TR signal on CW.
6. TR velocity profile.
7. Increase in tricuspid diastolic flow velocity (Vmax >0.8 m/s is significant).
8. Flow reversal on color Doppler of IVC and hepatic veins.
9. RA and RV cavity size and RV hypercontractility and abnormal septal motion.
10. Regurgitant fraction (see Chapter 10).

Pressure in the right atrium, right ventricle, and pulmonary artery

RAP (also see Chapter 2)

RVP and PAP systolic in mmHg (in absence of PS)

$$G + RAP = RVP = PAP\ (\text{systolic})$$

MPAP in mmHg

$$MPAP = 80 - 1/2\ AT$$

PAP diastolic (DPAP) in mmHg

$$DPAP = G + RVDP\ (\propto RAP)$$

REFERENCES

1. **Kostucki, W., Vandenbossche, J., Friart, A., and Englert, M.,** Pulsed Doppler regurgitant flow patterns of normal valves, *Am. J. Cardiol.,* 58, 309, 1986.
2. **Yock, P. G., Schnittger, I., and Popp, R. L.,** Is continuous wave Doppler too sensitive in diagnosing pathologic valvular regurgitation, *Circulation,* 70 (Suppl, II) (Abstr.), 381, 1984.
3. **Chopra, H.K., et al.,** Can color Doppler/two-dimensional echocardiography identify the need for tricuspid valve repair, *JACC,* 13(suppl A) (Abstr.), 24, 1989.
4. **Goldberg, S. J., Allen, H, D., Marx, G. R., and Donnerstein, R. L.,** *Doppler Echocardiography,* Lea and Febiger, Philadelphia, 1988.
5. **Dabestani, A., Mahan, G., Gardin, J., Takenaka, K., Burn, C., Alfie, A., and Henry, W,** Evaluation of pulmonary artery pressure and resistance by pulsed Doppler echocardiography, *Am. J. Cardiol.,* 59, 662, 1987.

ADDITIONAL READING

Suzuki, Y., et al., Detection and evaluation of tricuspid regurgitation using a real time, two-dimensional, color coded, Doppler flow imaging system: comparison with contrast two-dimensional echocardiogrpahy and right ventriculography, Am. J. Cardiol., 57, 811, 1986.

Hatle, L. and Angelsen, B. A., Non-invasive estimation of pulmonary artery systolic pressure with Doppler ultrasound, Br. Heart J., 45, 187, 1981.

Mahan, G., et al., Estimation of pulmonary artery pressure by pulsed Doppler echocardiography, *Circulation,* 68 (Suppl 3) (Abstr.), 367 1983.

Chapter 8

PROSTHETIC VALVES

I. DISCUSSION

As with native diseased valves, cardiac Doppler allows the assessment of prosthetic valves by determination of flow velocity profiles, the calculation of gradients ($4V^2$), the calculation of effective orifice areas, and the detection of valvular regurgitation. Comparative serial evaluations in the same patient are of particular value. Doppler, especially with color flow mapping, allows the detection of two or more flow profiles emanating from a prosthetic valve and allows differentiation of central vs. paravalvular regurgitant leaks. The importance of a baseline study, to allow a follow-up comparison study later, cannot be over-emphasized.

By echo-Doppler techniques one may assess the following characteristics of the various types of prosthetic valves and determine which are "normal" (or abnormal) for each type:

1. Range of velocities
2. Valve gradients
3. Pressure half-times (P1/2t)
4. Effective orifice areas
5. Regurgitation (valvular regurgitation is "normal" for some valves; paravalvular regurgitation is abnormal)

The above characteristics of the more common types of prosthetic valves have been published[1-6] and are summarized in the accompanying Figures 1 through 5.

In general, the normally functioning aortic prosthetic valve will have a *peak* systolic gradient of less than 45 mmHg. The normally functioning mitral prosthetic valve will usually have a *mean* diastolic gradient of less than 8 mmHg and a P1/2t of less than 170 ms.

In prosthetic valves that characteristically have two jets (e.g., Bjork-Shiley or Starr-Edwards in the mitral position), the velocities (as opposed to "size") in the two jets are usually quite similar and thus one can use either jet to obtain Vmax and other calculations. Also, it should be noted that in valves which should display two jets (Figure 6) the detection of only one usually indicates an abnormal valve.

It should be recalled that transient increases in prosthetic valve flow velocities and gradients in the early postoperative period may be due to an increase in flow and therefore allowances should be made in light of this observation. Also, velocity and gradient calculations for a few days following surgical commissurotomy or balloon valvuloplasty may be unreliable (probably due to

AORTIC PROSTHESIS (Mechanical)

Name	Peak Gradient (mmHg)	Mean Gradient (mmHg)	Patients with Mild AI
St. Jude	25.5 ± 5.1	12.5 ± 4.0	51%
Bjork–Shiley	23.8 ± 8.8	14.3 ± 5.2	22%
Starr–Edwards	38.6 ± 11.7	24.0 ± 4.0	52%

FIGURE 1. Doppler-determined characteristics for the normally functioning mechanical aortic valve prosthesis.

AORTIC PROSTHESIS (Tissue)

Name	Peak Gradient (mmHg)	Mean Gradient (mmHg)	Patients with Mild AI
Carpentier–Edwards	23.2 ± 8.7	14.4 ± 5.7	20%
Hancock	23.0 ± 6.7	11.0 ± 2.3	27%
Ionescu–Shiley	24.7 ± 7.6	14.0 ± 4.3	NA

FIGURE 2. Doppler-determined characteristics for the normally functioning tissue aortic valve prosthesis.

dynamic variation in size and compliance of reservoir and receiving chambers and changes in cardiac function).

Figure 7 presents a Doppler evaluation of a St. Jude prosthetic valve in the mitral position.

Tables 1 through 7 present "normal" (or abnormal) values for various prosthetic valves.

AORTIC PROSTHESIS (Influence of Size)

Name	Size	Peak Gradient (mmHg)	Mean Gradient (mmHg)
St. Jude	19	38 ± 20	22 ± 11
	21	26 ± 7	13 ± 5
	23	21 ± 12	10 ± 7
	25	20 ± 9	11 ± 6
Bjork–Shiley	21	30.5 ± 19.9	16
	23	27.3 ± 8.7	14 ± 5
	25	18.4 ± 5.3	13.3 ± 2.5
	27	14.6 ± 3.1	9.7 ± 2.5
Hancock	23	23.0 ± 4.6	12.0 ± 2
	25	20.7 ± 4.6	11.0 ± 2
	27	20.5 ± 5.7	10.0 ± 3
Carpentier – Edwards	21	27.3 ± 9.9	14.5 ± 6
	23	26.6 ± 8.9	12.7 ± 5.7
	25	24.4 ± 7.9	10.4 ± 2.3
	27	23.6 ± 7.2	9.9 ± 1

FIGURE 3. Influence of valve size on the Doppler-determined characteristics of various types of aortic valve prosthetic devices.

MITRAL PROSTHESIS (Mechanical)

Name	Peak Gradient (mmHg)	Mean Gradient (mmHg)	Mitral Valve Area (cm^2)	Patients with Mild MR
St. Jude	10.0 ± 3.6	3.5 ± 1.3	2.9 ± 0.6	30%
Bjork–Shiley	10.7 ± 2.7	2.9 ± 1.6	2.4 ± 0.6	16%
Starr–Edwards	14.6 ± 5.5	4.6 ± 2.4	2.0 ± 0.5	36%

FIGURE 4. Doppler-determined characteristics for the normally functioning mechanical mitral valve prosthesis.

MITRAL PROSTHESIS
(Tissue)

Name	Peak Gradient (mmHg)	Mean Gradient (mmHg)	Mitral Valve Area (cm^2)	Patients with Mild MR
Carpentier–Edwards	12.5 ± 3.6	6.5 ± 2.1	2.5 ± 0.7	NA
Hancock	9.7 ± 3.2	4.3 ± 2.1	1.7 ± 0.4	20%
Ionescu–Shiley	8.5 ± 2.9	3.3 ± 1.2	2.4 ± 0.8	NA

FIGURE 5. Doppler-determined characteristics for the normally functioning tissue mitral valve prosthesis.

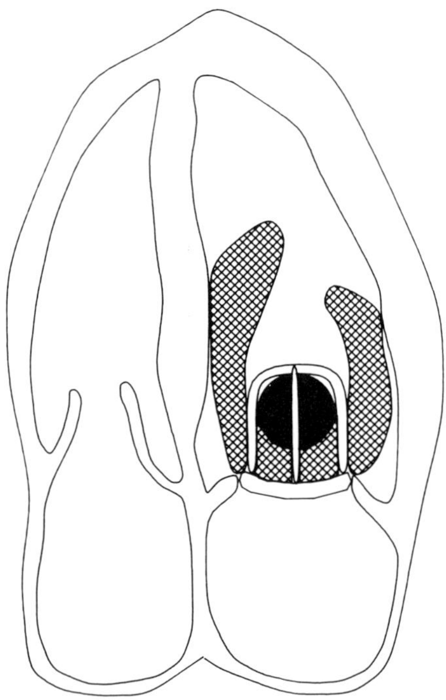

FIGURE 6. Artistic reproduction of a Doppler color-flow study of a Starr-Edwards prosthetic mitral valve, apical 4-chamber view, diastole. Note the characteristic double-flow profiles.

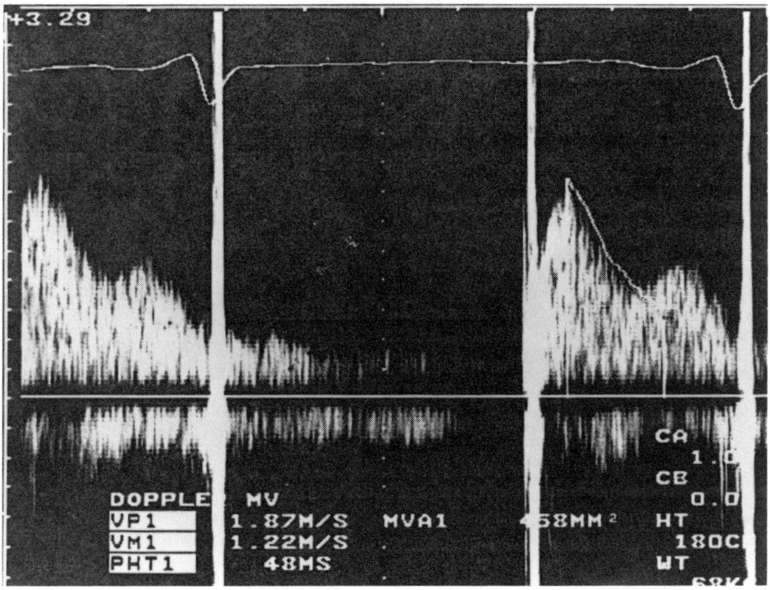

FIGURE 7. Continuous wave recording of diastolic flow velocity profile across a St. Jude prosthetic mitral valve. The peak velocity is 1.87 m/s. The calculated peak gradient [$4V^2 = 4(1.87)^2$] is 14 mmHg. The mean velocity is 1.22 m/s. The calculated mean gradient [$4V^2 = 4(1.22)^2$] is 5.95 mmHg. The P1/2t = 48 ms and the mitral valve area is 4.6 cm^2. From the accompanying Figure 4 it is evident these values are essentially normal for a St. Jude valve in the mitral position.

II. SUMMARY

Tables 1 through 7 present "normal" (or abnormal) values for various prosthetic valves.

Table 1
AORTIC PROSTHESIS
(MECHANICAL)

Name	Peak gradient (mmHg)	Mean gradient (mmHg)	Patients with mild AI %
St. Jude	25.5 ± 5.1	12.5 ± 6.3	51
Bjork-Shiley	23.8 ± 8.8	14.3 ± 5.2	22
Starr-Edwards	38.6 ± 11.7	24.0 ± 4.0	52

Table 2
AORTIC PROSTHESIS
(TISSUE)

Name	Peak gradient (mmHg)	Mean gradient (mmHg)	Patients with mild AI %
Carpentier-Edwards	23.2 ± 8.7	14.4 ± 5.7	20
Hancock	23.0 ± 6.7	11.0 ± 2.3	27
Ionescu-Shiley	24.7 ± 7.6	14.0 ± 4.3	N.A.

Note: N.A. = not available.

Table 3
AORTIC PROSTHESIS
(INFLUENCE OF SIZE)

Name	Size	Peak gradient (mmHg)	Mean gradient (mmHg)
St. Jude	19	38 ± 20	22 ± 11
	21	26 ± 7	13 ± 5
	23	21 ± 12	10 ± 7
	25	20 ± 9	11 ± 6
Bjork-Shiley	21	30.5 ± 19.9	16
	23	27.3 ± 8.7	14 ± 5
	25	18.4 ± 5.3	13.3 ± 2.5
	27	14.6 ± 3.1	9.7 ± 2.5
Hancock	23	23.0 ± 4.6	12.0 ± 2
	25	20.7 ± 4.6	11.0 ± 2
	27	20.5 ± 5.7	10.0 ± 3
Carpentier-Edwards	21	27.3 ± 9.9	14.5 ± 6
	23	26.6 ± 8.9	12.7 ± 5.7
	25	24.4 ± 7.9	10.4 ± 2.3
	27	23.6 ± 7.2	9.9 ± 1

Table 4
MITRAL PROSTHESIS (MECHANICAL)

Name	Peak gradient (mmHg)	Mean gradient (mmHg)	Mitral valve area (cm2)	Patients with mild MR %
St. Jude	10.0 ± 3.6	3.5 ± 1.3	2.9 ± 0.6	30
Bjork-Shiley	10.7 ± 2.7	2.9 ± 1.6	2.4 ± 0.6	16
Starr-Edwards	14.6 ± 5.5	4.6 ± 2.4	2.0 ± 0.5	36

Table 5
MITRAL PROSTHESIS (TISSUE)

Name	Peak gradient (mmHg)	Mean gradient (mmHg)	Mitral valve area (cm2)	Patients with mild MR %
Carpentier-Edwards	12.5 ± 3.6	6.5 ± 2.1	2.5 ± 0.7	N.A.
Hancock	9.7 ± 3.2	4.3 ± 2.1	1.7 ± 0.4	20
Ionescu-Shiley	8.5 ± 2.9	3.3 ± 1.2	2.4 ± 0.8	N.A.

Note: N.A. = not available.

REFERENCES

1. **Panidis, I. P., Ross, J., and Mintz, G. S.,** Normal and abnormal prosthetic valve function as assessed by Doppler echocardiography, *J. Am. Coll. Cardiol.,* 8, 317, 1986.
2. **Reisner, S. A. and Meltzer, R. S.,** Normal values of prosthetic valve Doppler echocardiographic parameters: a review, *J. Am. Soc. Echocardiol.,* 1, 201, 1988.
3. **Jacobs, L. E. and Kotler, M. N.,** Doppler echo evaluation of prosthetic valve function, *Cardiology,* July, 89, 1989.
4. **Burstow, D. J., et al.,** Continuous wave Doppler echocardiographic measurement of prosthetic valve gradients. A simultaneous Doppler-catheter correlative study, *Circulation,* 80, 50, 1989.
5. **Goldrath, N., Zimes, R., and Vered, Z.,** Analysis of Doppler-obtained velocity curves in functional evaluation of mechanical prosthetic valves in the mitral and aortic positions.
6. **Kapur, K. K., Fan, P., Nanda, N. C., et al.,** Doppler color flow mapping in the evaluation of prosthetic mitral and aortic valve function, *J. Am. Coll. Cardiol.,* 13, 1561, 1989.

ADDITIONAL READING

Wilkins, G. T., et al., Validation of continuous-wave Doppler echocardiographic measurements of mitral and tricuspid prosthetic valve gradients: A simultaneous Doppler-catheter study, *Circulation,* 74, 786, 1986.

Chapter 9

EVALUATION OF LEFT VENTRICULAR FUNCTION

I. SYSTOLIC FUNCTION

Evaluation of left ventricular (LV) global (vs. segmental) function may be accomplished by *M-mode echo* (our preferred formula is Teicholz)[1] or by *2-D echo* (our preferred formula is the modified Simpson)[2] calculating usually the LV stroke volume (SV), ejection fraction (EF) and cardiac output (CO). Cardiac *Doppler* may also be utilized to obtain measurements of global systolic LV function.

The Doppler method for obtaining the LV SV utilizes the formula:

$$SV = TVI \times A$$

where TVI is the time velocity integral (Chapter 4) of the LV systolic outflow profile and A is the area of the LV outflow tract (LVOT) or aortic root (AOR). The TVI is obtained by integrating the flow velocity curve or by the formula:

$$TVI = \text{Mean Vel} \times ET$$

where Mean Vel is the mean velocity calculated from the total systolic velocity profile obtained by continuous wave Doppler (CW) across the LVOT, the aortic valve and the AOR and ET is the ejection time. The mean velocity may be calculated manually but this determination is usually provided in the computer software of most modern equipment. An example of the aortic TVI is shown in Figure 1.

The area (A) of the LVOT is calculated from the diameter (d) of the LVOT as determined in the 2-D parasternal long-axis view, measured in midsystole from the point where the base of the anterior (right) aortic cusp meets the interventricular septum to the point where the base of the posterior (non-coronary) aortic cusp meets the base of the anterior mitral valve leaflet (Figure 2). The d of the AOR may be measured from the M-mode echo or from the 2-D echo study (measured in the AOR just above the tips of the aortic cusps). Either way, the formula then is

$$A = \pi r^2 = 3.14 \times \left(\frac{d}{2}\right)^2 = cm^2$$

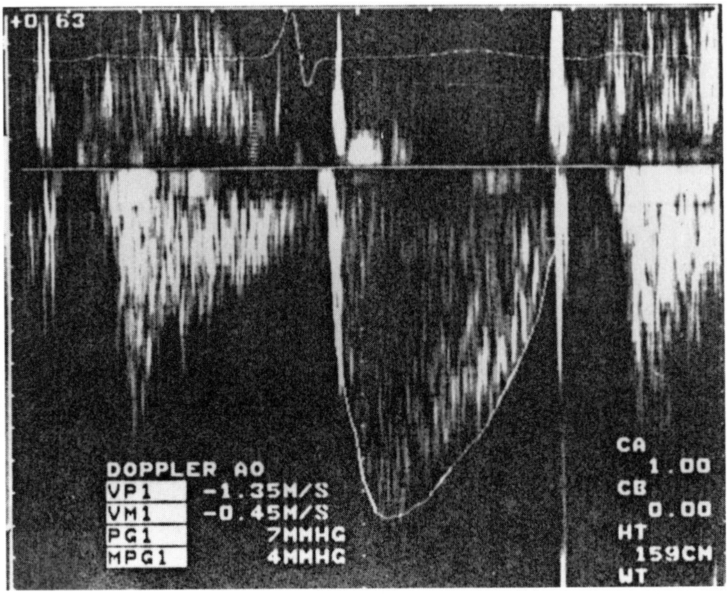

FIGURE 1. CW recording across the LVOT, the aortic valve, and aortic root during systole. Note a peak velocity (Vmax) measured at 1.35 m/s (normal value). Note the equipment computer calculation of the mean velocity at 0.45 m/s (45 cm/s). The horizontal time markers (top of illustration) are at 100 ms. The aortic flow velocity curve occurs over a time (ejection time, ET) of 318 ms (0.318 s). Therefore, the aortic TVI (TVIa) is

$$\text{TVIa} = \text{mean Vel} \times \text{ET}$$

$$45 \text{ cm/s} \times 0.318 \text{ s}$$

$$\text{TVIa} = 14.31 \text{ cm}$$

Thus,

$$\text{SV} = \text{TVI (cm)} \times \text{A} \left(\text{cm}^2\right) = \text{cm}^3 \text{ (cc)}$$

$$\text{SV} = \frac{\text{cc}}{1000} = \text{l (liters)}$$

and

$$\text{CO} = \text{SV} \times \text{HR} = \text{l/min}$$

where CO is cardiac output and HR is heart rate (beats per minute). An example of this calculation of the LV CO is given based on data from Figures 1 and 2.

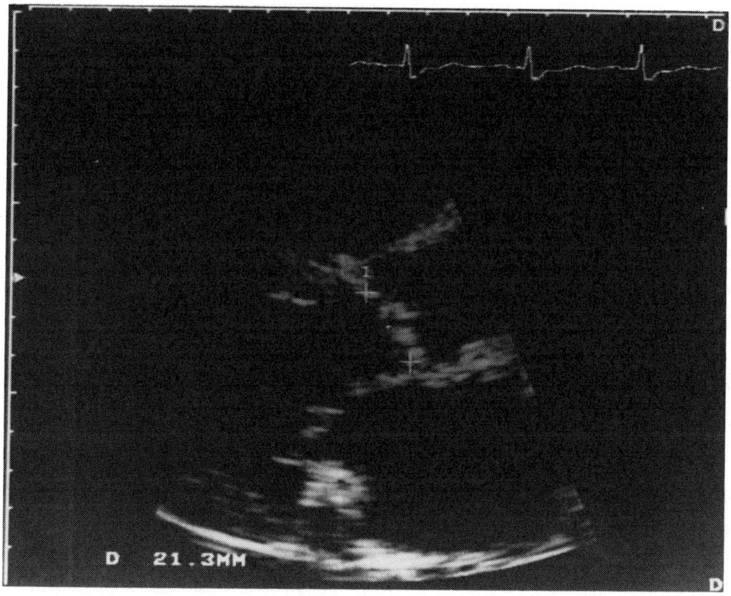

FIGURE 2. 2-D parasternal long-axis view of aortic root, aortic valve, interventricular septum, and anterior mitral valve. The diameter of the LVOT is measured between the markers (+) as 21.3 mm (2.13 cm). The area (A) of the LVOT is then

$$A = \pi r^2 = 3.14 \times \left(\frac{d}{2}\right)^2$$
$$= 3.14 \times \left(\frac{2.13}{2}\right)^2$$
$$A = 3.56 \text{ cm}^2$$

Thus,

$$SV = TVI_a \text{ (cm)} \times A \left(\text{cm}^2\right) = \text{cm}^3 \text{ (cc)}$$
$$= 14.31 \times 3.56$$
$$SV = 50.94 \text{ cc}$$
$$SV = \frac{50.94}{1000} = 0.0511 \text{ (liters)}$$

Then CO at HR of 90 BPM would be

$$CO = SV \times HR = \text{l/min}$$
$$= 0.051 \times 90$$
$$CO = 4.59 \text{ l/min}$$

The LV end-diastolic volume (EDV) may be determined by M-mode or 2-D echo methods and SV by Doppler, then:

$$EF = \frac{SV}{EDV} \times 100 = \text{ejection fraction } \%$$

As noted above, we prefer the Teicholz formula for determination of LV volume by M-mode echo since this method attempts to correct for changes in geometric shapes as heart sizes change. The formula is

$$V = \left[\frac{7.0}{2.4 + LVID}\right] LVID^3$$

where V is LV volume and LVID is LV internal dimension. The dimensions for systole and diastole are substituted in the equation and end-systolic volume (ESV) and EDV are calculated. Thus,

$$SV = EDV - ESV$$

$$CO = SV \times HR$$

$$EF = \frac{EDV - ESV}{EDV} \times 100 = \%$$

LV volumes may be determined from the 2-D echo study. We prefer the modified Simpson formula which is

$$EDV = \frac{LVLD}{9} \times \left(4 \times LVAMD + 2 \times LVAPD + \sqrt{LVAMD \times LVAPD}\right)$$

$$ESV = \frac{LVLS}{9} \times \left(4 \times LVAMS + 2 \times LVAPS + \sqrt{LVAMS \times LVAPS}\right)$$

where LVLD (or LVLS) is LV length measured in a long-axis view from the LV apex to mitral annulus level in diastole (and systole), LVAMD (or LVAMS) is the LV area measured at the mitral valve level in diastole (and systole), and LVAPD (or LVAPS) is the LV area measured at the papillary muscle level in diastole (and systole).

Figure 3 (A, B, and C) illustrates the utilization of the modified Simpson rule in the determination of standard LV systolic functions.

The above calculations will be important in formulations to evaluate regurgitant fractions (Chapter 10).

A. OTHER PARAMETERS OF LEFT VENTRICULAR (LV) SYSTOLIC FUNCTION

For many years, a number of hemodynamic measurements derived at cardiac catheterization have been utilized as indices of LV systolic function. Among the most popular of these have been (1) peak systolic aortic blood flow

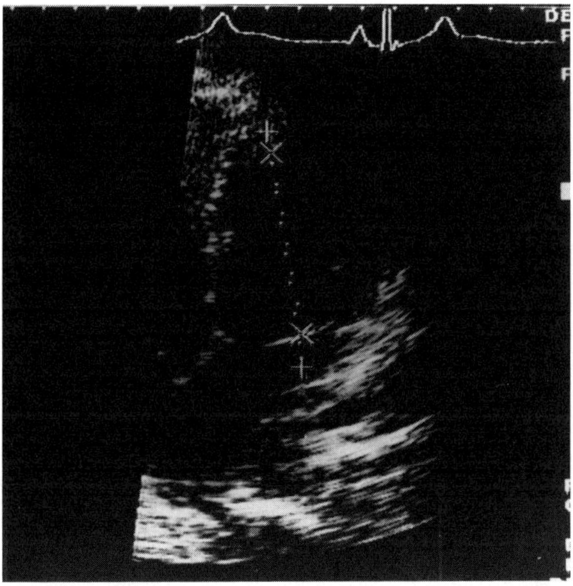

A

FIGURE 3. (A) *Modified Simpson formula:* illustration of determination of LV length in systole (X) (LVLS) and diastole (+) (LVLD) from the LV endocardial apex to mitral annulus is an apical 4-chamber view. (B) *Modified* Simpson formula: illustration of measurement and calculation of LV area at the mitral valve level measured in systole (LVAMS) and diastole (LVAMD). (C) Modified Simpson formula: illustration of measurement and calculation of LV area at the papillary muscle level measured in systole (LVAPS) and diastole (LVAPD). From the above values the equipment computer calculated the following: EDV = 133.8 ml, ESV = 50.0 ml, SV = 83.8 ml, CO = 4.27 l/min, and EF = 0.63 = 63%.

velocity, (2) mean aortic blood flow acceleration, and (3) maximal aortic blood flow acceleration.

A recent publication by Isaaz et al.[3] has shown that maximal aortic blood flow acceleration is closely related to the maximal force exerted by the LV in early systole and that an EF index (which may be readily determined by Doppler study) appears more accurate than peak aortic blood flow velocity and mean aortic blood flow acceleration for the assessment of systolic LV function. As noted,[3] *force* is a well-established physical term, which, according to Newton's second law of motion, is defined as the product of mass and acceleration, i.e., force = mass × acceleration. The unit of force is a dyne which is the amount of force that imparts to a mass of 1.0 g an acceleration of 1.0 cm per second per second.

Recall that Doppler-determined volume relates to velocity (TVI, see Chapter 4) × area. Volume flow then relates to this volume flowing over a given

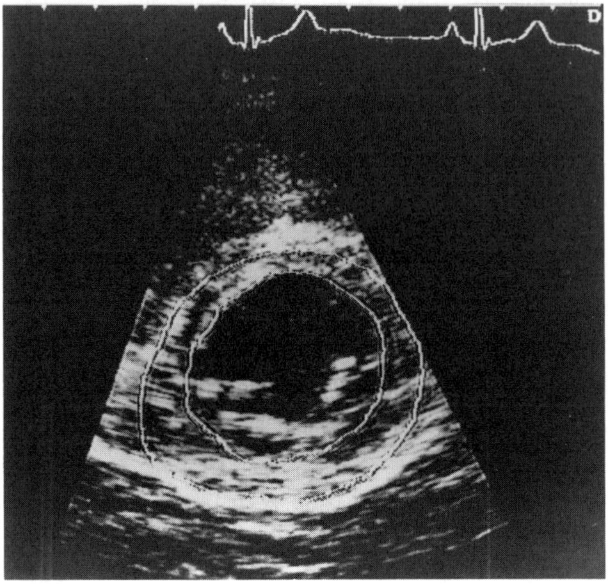

FIGURE 3B

period of time. Blood volume (Vol) may be converted to mass (M) by:

$$M = Vol \times p$$

where p is the mass density of blood (1.06 g/cm^3).

As indicated above, aortic or LV outflow area (A) is calculated from the aortic annular diameter (d) measured on 2-D echo immediately proximal to the insertion points of the aortic leaflets during early systole as:

$$A = \pi r^2 = \pi\left(\frac{d}{d}\right)^2 = 3.14\left(\frac{d}{2}\right)^2$$

Other pertinent factors for the calculation of the force index are illustrated in Figure 4. In this figure note the LV systolic outflow velocity curve. This may be determined by pulsed Doppler with the sample volume placed first into the aortic valve leaflets then gradually moved backward toward the apex until the first clear ventricular outflow velocity is obtained. Any further apical movement of the sample volume would result in a reduction in velocity. The optimal flow pattern is evident by finding the highest recorded velocity with the least spectral dispersion. As usual, the velocity curve is analyzed by following the contour of the darkest portion of the curve (generally analyzing 4 to 6 cardiac cycles and taking an average of the measurements). In the absence of aortic

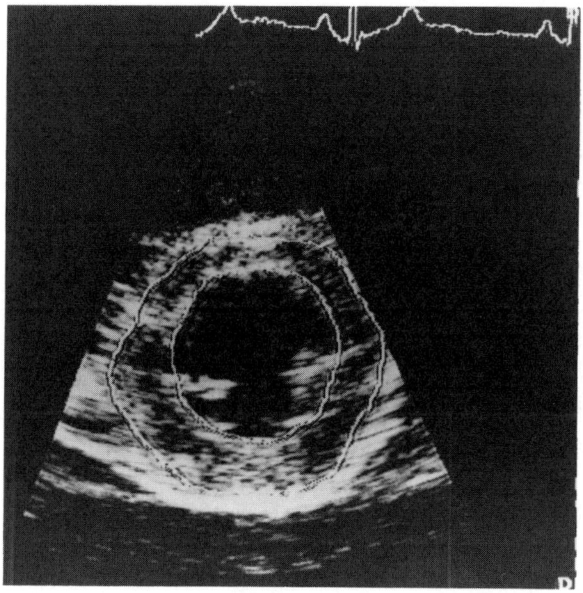

FIGURE 3C

stenosis, CW might be utilized in these determinations; although, in general, for the LV force calculations, patients with significant aortic and mitral valve disease should probably be excluded. In the illustration, note a peak velocity (PkV) of 1.1 m/s (110 cm/s) and an acceleration time of 100 ms (0.1 s).

Since the flow velocities of interest in the force calculations occur during the acceleration time (AT) of the velocity curve, then the TVI would be that occurring during this period of time, TVI_{AT} (shaded area in the figure).

It is of interest that the left ventricle contributes little to ejection during late systole. In late systole, after the positive acceleration is over (and maximal velocity has been attained) the blood continues to flow under its own momentum until resistance stops it. Thus, LV ejection force determined during early systole (acceleration time) appears to be conceptually appropriate to assess LV systolic function. Also, it appears that early systolic flow is much less influenced by changes in preload than flow during late systole.

As noted by formulations reviewed before:

$$\text{Blood volume} = \text{TVI} \times \text{A}$$

Converting volume to mass (M) with this mass moving over the AT gives:

$$M_{AT} = p \times TVI_{AT} \times CSA$$

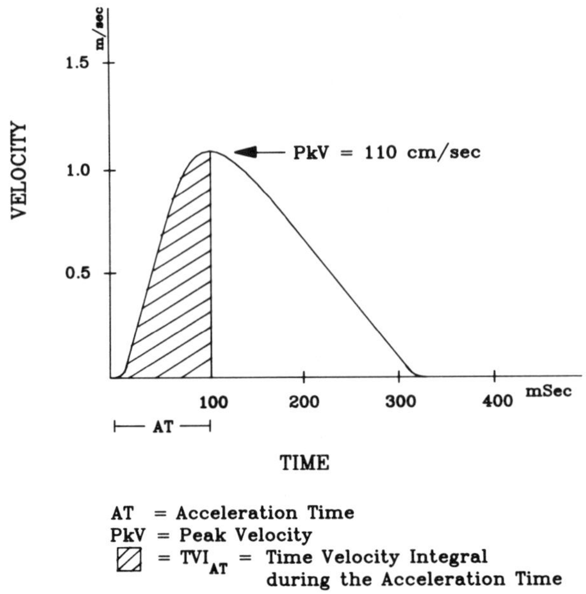

FIGURE 4. Illustrations of a CW or pulsed wave Doppler recording of the flow velocity profile of the LVOT during systole.

where CSA is the cross-sectional area of the aortic annulus or LVOT.

The average acceleration (AA) undergone during the AT is

$$AA = \frac{PkV}{t} = cm/s/s$$

where PkV is the peak velocity and t is the AT.

Thus, in review,

$$\text{Force} = \text{Mass} \times \text{acceleration}$$

and mass during acceleration is

$$M_{AT} = p \times TVI_{AT} \times CSA$$

and mean or AA is

$$AA = \frac{PkV}{t}$$

Therefore, mean ejection force (MEF, dynes) during the acceleration time (MEF_{AT}) is

$$MEF_{AT} = \underbrace{p \times TVI_{AT} \times CSA}_{M_{AT}} \times \underbrace{\frac{PkV}{t}}_{AA} = \text{dynes}$$

and,

$$\frac{\text{dynes}}{1000} = \text{K dynes}$$

An example of the application of these formulations as based on Figure 4 would be as follows:

$$p = 1.06\ \text{g/cm}^3$$
$$TVI_{AT} = 5.5\ \text{cm (shaded portion of curve)}$$
$$d = 2.0\ \text{cm (measured diameter of the aortic annulus)}$$
$$CSA = 3.14 \times \left(\frac{d}{2}\right)^2 = 3.14\ \text{cm}^2$$
$$PkV = 1.1\ \text{m/s} = 110\ \text{cm/s}$$
$$t = AT = 100\ \text{m sec} = 0.1\ \text{s}$$

Thus:

$$\begin{aligned} M_{AT} &= p \times TVI_{AT} \times CSA \\ &= \frac{1.06\ \text{g}}{\text{cm}^3} \times 5.5\ \text{cm} \times 3.14\ \text{cm}^2 \\ &= 1.06\ \text{g} \times 5.5 \times 3.14 \\ &= 18.2\ \text{g} \end{aligned}$$

and:

$$\begin{aligned} AA &= \frac{PkV}{t} \\ &= \frac{110\ \text{cm/s}}{0.1\ \text{s}} \\ &= 1100\ \text{cm/s} \end{aligned}$$

Finally:

or

$$\text{Force} = \text{Mass} \times \text{acceleration}$$

or

$$\begin{aligned} MEF_{AT} &= M_{AT} \times AA = \text{dynes} \\ &= 18.2 \times 1100 \\ &= 20020 \text{ dynes} = 20.20 \text{ K dynes} \end{aligned}$$

Figure 5 illustrates the integration (TVI) during the AT from an actual recording of an LVOT systolic flow velocity curve. This provides the TVI_{AT} which the equipment computer determines in this instance to be 0.06 m or 6.0 cm.

Normal values for the LV systolic outflow parameters noted above were given as:

Peak velocity (cm/s)	108 ± 7
Mean (average) acceleration (cm/s/s)	1209 ± 282
Accelerated blood mass (g)	25 ± 6
Ejection force (K dynes)	29 ± 5
Ejection force/BSA (K dynes/m²)	17 ± 3

Of interest, the values determined for a group of patients with *chronic congestive heart failure* (with cardiac catheterization-derived LV ejection fractions of ≤40%) were given as:[3]

Peak velocity (cm/s)	73 ± 14
Mean (average) acceleration (cm/s/s)	684 ± 117
Accelerated blood mass (g)	17 ± 4
Ejection force (K dynes)	12 ± 4
Ejection force/BSA (K dynes/M²)	7 ± 2

In general, a mean LV ejection force less than 20 K dynes is associated with a depressed LV performance (ejection fraction <50%) with a 91% sensitivity and 90% specificity.[3]

These differences between normals and patients with congestive heart failure (ejection fraction ≤40%) were obviously highly significant and, of importance, statistically significant differences were maintained in chronic congestive heart failure patients even with EF of 41 to 60%, a group in which peak velocity and mean acceleration values did not differ from normals. The higher accuracy of force data in the assessment of LV function probably lies in the fact that *acceleration* is only one of the two terms of *force,* the second term being the *mass.* As indicated,[3] to assess LV ejection dynamics more appropriately, both terms should be considered according to the basic mass–acceleration concept. Clearly, a greater mass requires a greater force than would a smaller mass to undergo the same acceleration, thereby implying a higher level of cardiac performance. It appears that peak aortic blood velocity and mean acceleration are maintained within normal limits as long as severe LV function

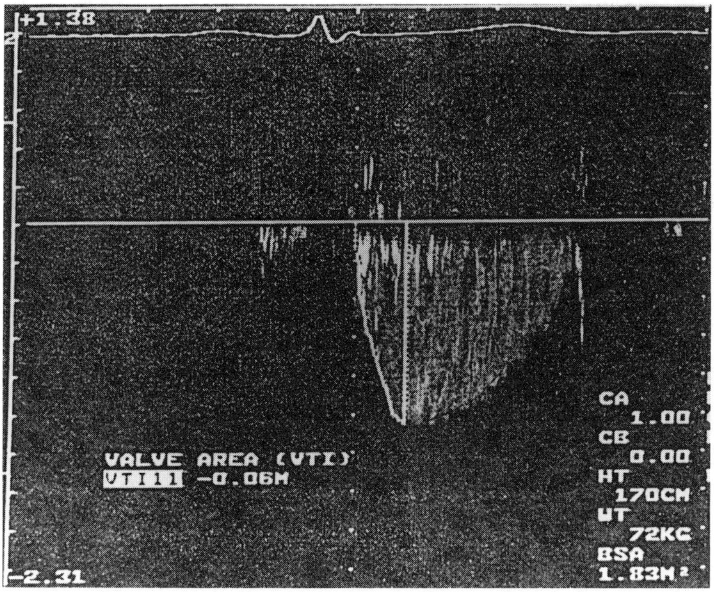

FIGURE 5. CW systolic LVOT velocity flow curve illustrating the integration (TVI) during the acceleration time (AT) of this curve. This provides the TVI_{AT} which in this instance is 0.06 m or 6.0 cm. This illustration is artistically retouched for clarification.

does not occur. The mean LV ejection force is more sensitive for the diagnosis of mild to moderate LV dysfunction.

The validity of the above detailed LV systolic force determinations has been supported by a recent study documenting impairment of this function in patients with hypothyroidism.[4]

II. DIASTOLIC FUNCTION

Mitral diastolic flow velocities and patterns are generally easy to record (pulsed Doppler is the preferred means for diastolic function evaluation). It is reasonable to assume that mitral diastolic flow velocity patterns reflect rates of change of volume flowing into the LV,[5] this result being dependent upon the temporal and quantitative changes in the left atrial (LA) to LV diastolic pressure gradients. A recent excellent review of the subject of Doppler evaluation of LV diastolic function[6] details the many complexities encountered in these evaluations, however. Unfortunately, changes in mitral diastolic flow velocities may vary significantly with factors other than changes in LV diastolic function. These include changes in loading conditions (preload and afterload), differing heart rates, cardiac arrhythmias, heart blocks and AV dissociations, presence of valvular abnormalities, and changes in atrial and ventricular contractile states.

Under ideal conditions, with all variables controlled, the typical transmitral diastolic flow pattern is as depicted in Figure 6. Note the peak early diastolic filling (E), the peak late diastolic filling following atrial contraction (A), the acceleration time (AT), and the deceleration time (DT) of the early diastolic flow pattern. Typically, impairment in LV filling and a decrease in LV compliance would produce a flow pattern as depicted in Figure 7. Note a slight slowing in the AT, a greater slowing in the DT, a lower peak E, a higher peak A, and a decrease in the E:A ratio.

Regarding the above measurements, an increase in LV afterload causes a decrease in transmitral diastolic peak velocity and a prolongation of the DT. Also, preload reduction causes a decrease in early peak velocity and a prolongation of DT. Increase in preload (e.g., fluid loading) causes an increase in peak velocities and a shortening of the DT.[6] With an increase in heart rate or prolongation of the PR interval (or both), the E and A velocities may merge to form a single waveform in diastole.[6] Atrial flutter and fibrillation and any form of AV dissociation causes considerable difficulty in obtaining meaningful diastolic measurements. Severe aortic valvular insufficiency causes a rapid decrease in the gradient between the left atrium (LA) and LV and, therefore, the mitral E waveform will show a rapid DT. In severe mitral regurgitation, the presence of a large "V" wave in the LA pressure raises the LA-LV gradient and the mitral initial peak velocity (E) will be high.[6]

Some of these complex relationships may be more easily understood by mechanisms as simplistically depicted in Figure 8 through 16. Recall the formula:

$$F = V \times A$$

where F is flow, V is velocity (or TVI), and A is area (through which the flow moves). Regarding transmitral diastolic flow, if diastolic flow time (cycle length) is constant and mitral valve area is constant, then:

$$F\,(cc) = V\,(cm/s)$$

In these circumstances, therefore, the velocity (cm/s) for "E" and for "A" represent the flow during those times in the cardiac cycle. Although LV diastolic processes are extremely complex (e.g., active LV relaxation is an energy-dependent process; energy is required to move calcium from the actin-myosin complex back to the sarcoplasmic reticulum), for practical purposes LV filling may be viewed as involving two functions. One is the early passive filling following the opening of the mitral valve (E-wave) and the other is late

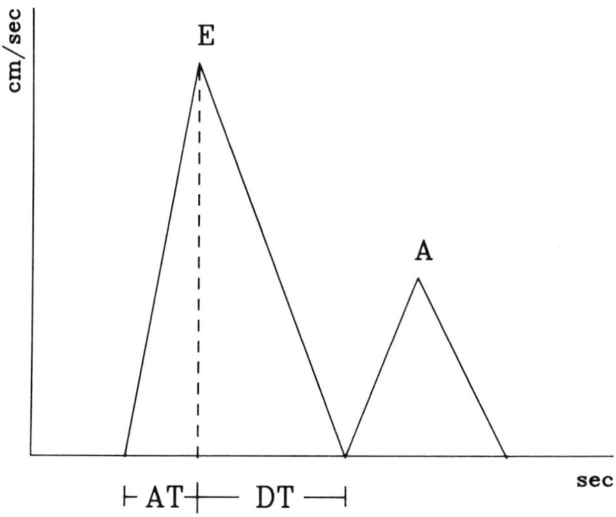

FIGURE 6. Diagram of "typical" normal transmitral diastolic flow pattern (usually by pulsed wave Doppler). AT = acceleration time. DT = deceleration time. E and A waves noted.

diastolic filling during LA contraction (A-wave). The mitral valve may be considered as a "flow gate" and the E-wave and A-wave as reflections of the temporal and quantitative change in LA-LV gradient. The effects of varying "loading" conditions combined with changes in LV diastolic compliance can then be schematically illustrated (Figures 8 to 16). The LA is considered a reservoir reflecting "preload filling pressure". The MV opens and fills the LV in large part by "passive" mechanisms (E) and then to a smaller degree by atrial contraction (A). In Figure 8 the LA reservoir is represented at 140 cc, the LV end-systolic volume (ESV) at 70 cc, the early LV passive filling at 80 cc, the atrial contraction contribution to LV filling at 20 cc, the LV end-diastolic volume (EDV) at 170 cc, and the LV stroke volume (SV) to occur during the following systole at 100 cc. In this highly simplified illustration, the EF then would be

$$\frac{\text{EDV} - \text{ESV}}{\text{EDV}} \times 100 = \text{EF\%}$$

$$\frac{170 - 70}{170} \times 100 = 59\%$$

The "compliant" and "noncompliant" LV flow patterns are depicted in Figures 8 through 10 under normal "loading" conditions. With the "noncompliant" LV as illustrated in Figures 9 and 10B, the atrial contraction (A)

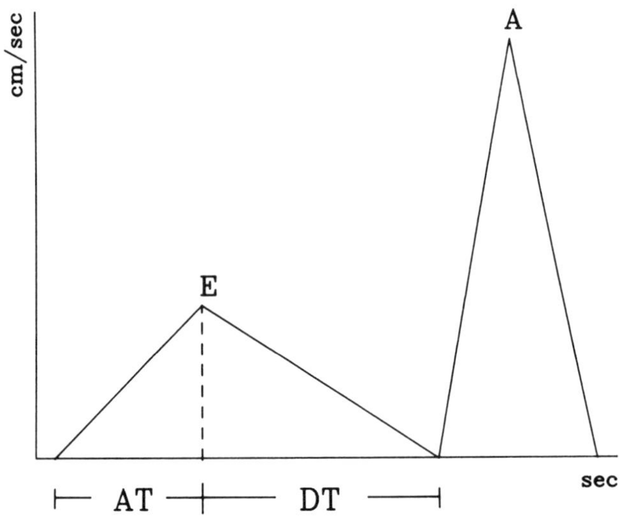

FIGURE 7. Diagram of a "typical" transmitral diastolic flow pattern in a patient with abnormal (decreased) LV compliance.

contribution to LV filling must "make up" for that blood which the "stiff" LV could not accept during early passive filling (E), specifically if a stable CO is to be maintained. Similar consideration as in Figures 8 through 10 may be given to Figures 11 through 13 for enhanced, and Figures 14 to 16 for reduced, "loading" conditions, respectively. Note that the filling patterns (E and A) for the same "noncompliant" LV as illustrated in Figure 10B may be converted to "normal" filling patterns (E and A) by increasing preload (Figure 13B). An example of this phenomenon in clinical practice occurs during the late states ("burned out") of a hypertrophic cardiomyopathy when congestive heart failure (increased preload) develops (even with little or no significant change in LV diastolic compliance).

In light of the above, the following points appear to be clear: (1) if "loading" conditions (and other factors as mentioned) are stable, the E-wave, A-wave, E/A ratio, AT of E-wave, and DT of E wave all relate closely to changes in LV diastolic compliance, and (2) if LV compliance (and other factors as mentioned) is stable then the above-noted waveforms relate closely to changes in loading conditions.

Qualitative "corrections" relative to the above may be attempted by Doppler assessment of "preload" conditions (e.g., PA systolic, mean, and diastolic pressures) (see Chapter 7). "Afterload" conditions, of course, may be assessed by arterial blood pressure measurement, CO, EF, and peripheral vascular resistance.

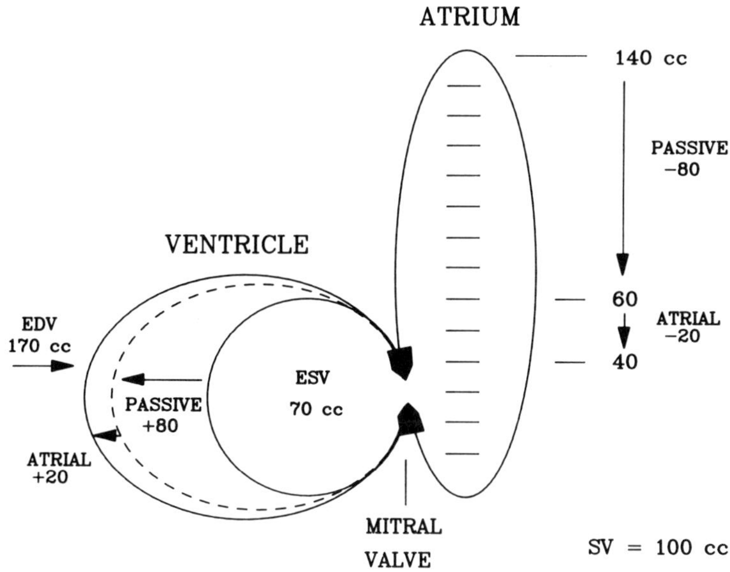

FIGURE 8. Diastolic function with a compliant LV, normal loading conditions: schematic representation of the left atrium (LA) and left ventricle (LV). The LA is represented as a reservoir of 140 cc. After the mitral valve opens the LA "passively" loses 80 cc which it contributes to the LV filling. With atrial contraction the LA "actively" contributes another 20 cc to LV filling (a total of 100 cc). The LV end systolic volume (ESV) is depicted at 70 cc. After the mitral valve opens, it "passively" receives 80 cc from the LA (thus producing the Doppler recorded "E" wave, Figure 10A) and, with atrial contraction, the LV "actively" receives another 20 cc from the LA (thus producing the Doppler recorded "A" wave, Figure 10A).

There is considerable variation in the literature for suggested "normal values" relative to the above-noted parameters of mitral diastolic flow velocities and patterns. These differences are probably explained by differences in population groups studied and by variations in Doppler technique (e.g., spatial placement of the pulsed Doppler sample volume in different areas of the mitral apparatus and variation in measurement lines and points along the mitral diastolic velocity display) along with other factors as noted above. Values from one study[7] of transmitral diastolic flow are as follows:

Peak E (cm/s)	86 ± 16
Peak A (cm/s)	56 ± 13
Ratio E:A	1.6 ± 0.5
AT (m/s)	73 ± 10
DT (m/s)	199 ± 32

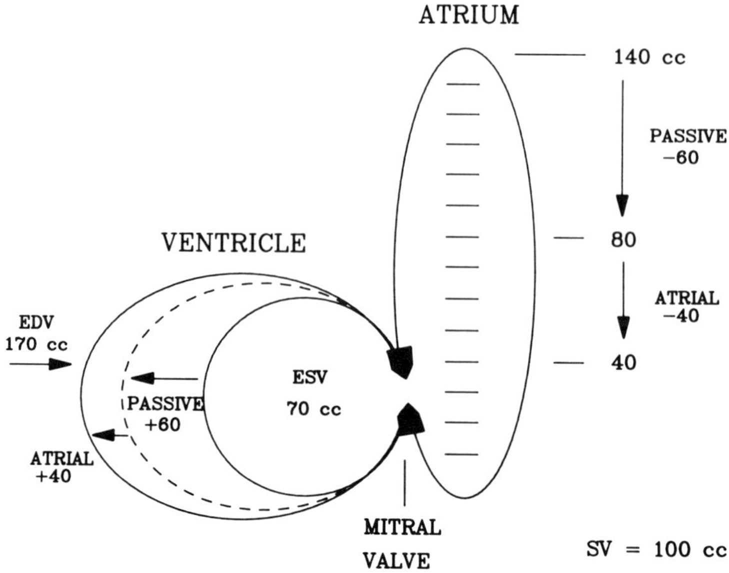

FIGURE 9. LV diastolic function, noncompliant LV, normal loading conditions: in this situation, the noncompliant LV can receive only 60 cc passively from the LA (thus the Doppler derived "E" wave diminishes, Figure 10B) but to sustain proper LV filling (for subsequent normal LV systolic function) the LA must contribute more during contraction, 40 cc in this instance, (thus the Doppler derived "A" wave is increased, Figure 10B).

Normal values published in a more recent study[8] are as follows:

Peak E (cm/s)	66 ± 13
Peak A (cm/s)	45 ± 5
Ratio E:A	1.5 ± 0.3
E area (M)	0.094 ± 0.022
A area (M)	0.034 ± 0.007
Total area (M)	0.126 ± 0.026
*E area/A area	2.7 ± 0.51
*A area/total area	0.28 ± 0.04
Peak E/total area	5.23 ± 1.7

In the above study it was of interest that reduction in LV compliance secondary to ischemia due to significant proximal stenosis in the left anterior descending artery (as compared to normals) was indicated best by the *E area/A area ($p < 0.001$) and *A area/total area ($p < 0.001$). The area measurements represented areas under the time-velocity curve of the mitral inflow (TVI, see Chapter 4).

Until recently, it was thought that the most practical and accurate means to

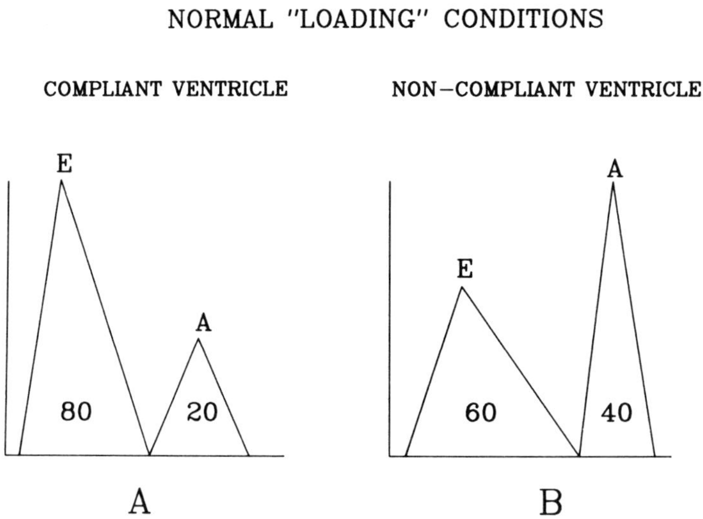

FIGURE 10. Diagrammatic representation of the Doppler-derived transmitral diastolic filling pattern under normal loading conditions. Figure 10A, compliant LV. Figure 10B, noncompliant LV. Note the total cubic centimeters transported from the LA to the LV is the same in each instance, but the pattern (temporal and volumetric) of filling is markedly different. Note how the "abnormal" pattern in Figure 10B could be changed to a "normal" filling pattern (Figure 13B) simply by increasing the loading (preload) conditions.

assess LV diastolic function noninvasively was to utilize radionuclide-derived peak filling rates, particularly those normalized to LV EDV. By convention, radionuclide peak filling rate was normalized to EDV to derive a filling *index* that eliminated errors involved in converting counts to absolute volumes. An extremely attractive counterpart of this type of analysis, as might be applied to cardiac Doppler studies, was recently published.[9]

Doppler echocardiography has the ability to measure peak filling rate but application of these techniques has been limited by technical errors in quantitative echocardiographic determination of mitral annulus cross-sectional area (flow = velocity × area) and ventricular volumes (i.e., to "normalize"). Normalization of Doppler peak filling rate to mitral SV[9] rather than EDV permits the derivation of a diastolic filling index relatively free of errors caused by geometric assumptions (eg., annulus as a circle), diameter measurements, and sample volume positioning (minor variations which may significantly influence flow velocities and patterns).

Normalization to mitral SV allows the derivation of a Doppler *peak filling index* that is calculated entirely from mitral inflow velocity and is therefore independent of diameter measurements and geometric assumptions.[9]

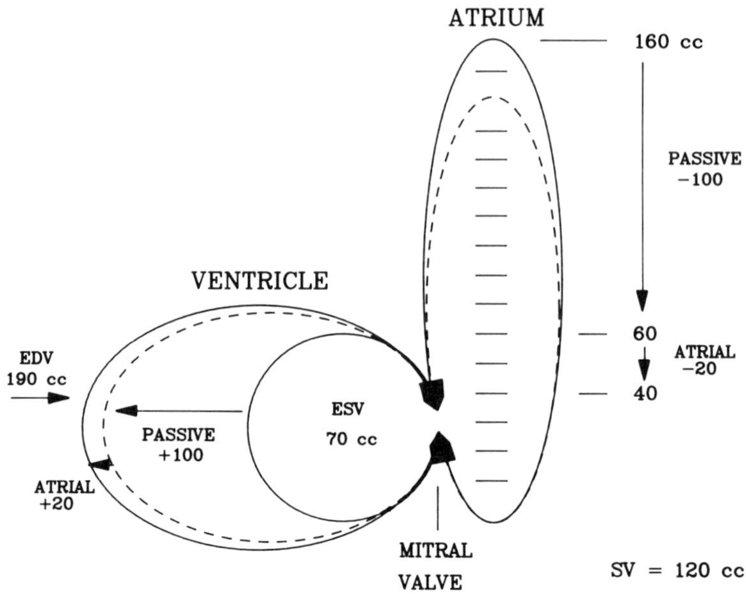

FIGURE 11. LV diastolic function, *enhanced* loading (preload) conditions, *compliant* LV. This results in a mitral diastolic filling pattern depicted in Figure 13A.

Thus, PFR (cc/s) = LV peak filling rate in cc/s; V (cm/s) = early peak filling velocity in cm/s (E); MAA (cm^2) = mitral valve annulus area in cm^2. Flow = velocity × area; and PFR (cc/s) = V (cm/s) × MAA (cm^2).

To derive the peak filling rate normalized to mitral SV, the absolute peak filling rate is divided by the mitral SV.[7]

Thus,

$$\text{PFR}\left(\text{sv/s}\right)=\frac{\text{V}\left(\text{cm/s}\right)\times\text{MAA}\left(\text{cm}^2\right)}{\text{SV}\left(\text{cc}\right)}$$

$$\text{SV}\left(\text{cc}\right)=\text{TV Im}\left(\text{cm}\right)\times\text{MAA}\left(\text{cm}^2\right)$$

TVI = mean velocity × mitral diastolic filling time (or by planimetry).

Therefore:

$$\text{PFR}\left(\text{sv/s}\right)=\frac{\text{V}\left(\text{cm/s}\right)\times\text{MAA}\left(\text{cm}^2\right)}{\text{TVIm}\ \left(\text{cm}\right)\times\text{MAA}\left(\text{cm}^2\right)}$$

or

$$\text{PFR}\left(\text{sv/s}\right)=\frac{\text{V}\left(\text{cm/s}\right)}{\text{TV Im}\left(\text{cm}\right)}=\text{Index}$$

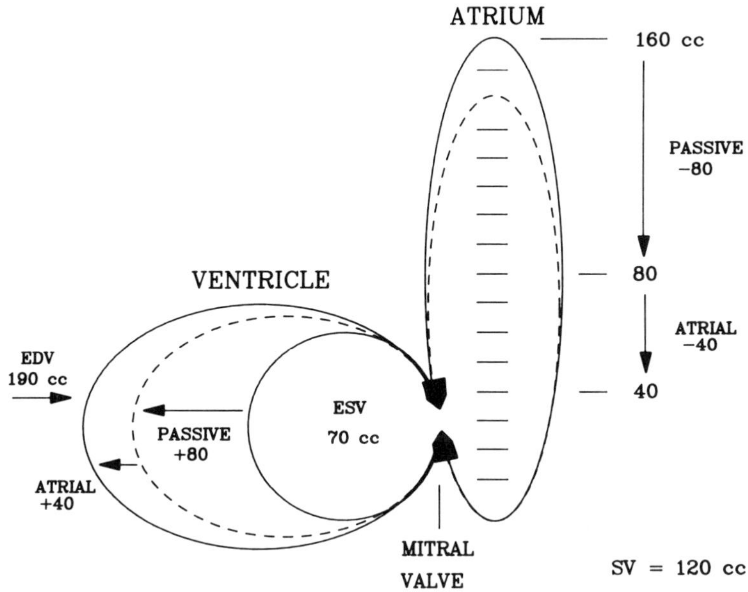

FIGURE 12. LV diastolic functions, *enhanced* loading (preload) conditions, *non-compliant* LV. This results in a mitral diastolic filling pattern depicted in Figure 13B.

Normal index values given were[9]

$$PFR = 5.06 + 1.6$$

It should be noted that the mitral E:A ratio increases significantly (∝50%) when the pulsed Doppler sample volume moves from the annulus (the site commonly sampled) to the tips of the mitral leaflets. As opposed to the E:A ratio, the normalized PFR (sv/s) does not change whether the pulsed Doppler sample volume is at the annulus or at the tips of the mitral leaflets.[9] Finally, the normalized PFR may alleviate some of the problems encountered in varying LV loading conditions (as discussed earlier).

Recall that an important precondition to the use of Doppler transmitral waveforms and flow for assessing diastolic function is the absence of valvular abnormalities that may alter ventricular filling, such as mitral stenosis, severe mitral regurgitation (increased diastolic flow), and severe aortic regurgitation (impedes mitral diastolic filling). The normalized PFR may prove to be of value even in these situations.

Figure 17 illustrates the mitral peak filling rate normalized to mitral SV in a patient with reduced LV compliance.

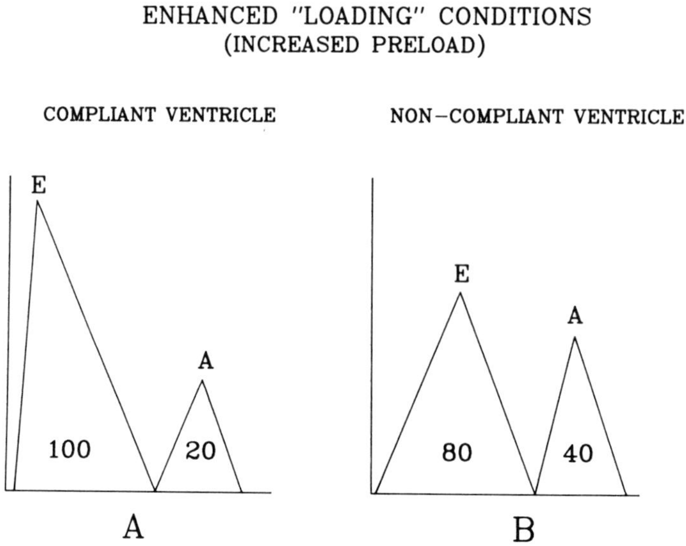

FIGURE 13. Mitral diastolic filling patterns under *enhanced* loading (preload) conditions. Figure 13A is a compliant LV, Figure 13B is a noncompliant LV. Note how a "normal" filling pattern in Figure 13B could be altered to reflect an "abnormal" filling due to a noncompliant ventricle, simply by reducing loading (preload) conditions to normal (Figure 10B).

A. LV MASS

Left ventricular (LV) mass may be calculated by the formula measured best from 2-D-guided M-mode study.

$$\text{LV mass} = 1.04\ [(\text{LVID}_d + \text{LVPW}_d + \text{IVS}_d)^3] - (\text{LVID}_d)^3] - 13.6$$

where LVID_d = LV internal diameter in diastole (cm), LVPW_d = LV posterior wall thickness in diastole (cm), and IVS_d = interventricular wall thickness in diastole (cm).

$$\text{LV mass Index} = \frac{\text{LV mass}}{\text{BSA}}$$

Normal values are:

LV mass (Gm)	
Men	80 – 210
Women	75 – 150

$$\text{LV mass Index} = 92 \pm 16\ \text{Gm}/\text{M}^2\ \text{BSA}$$

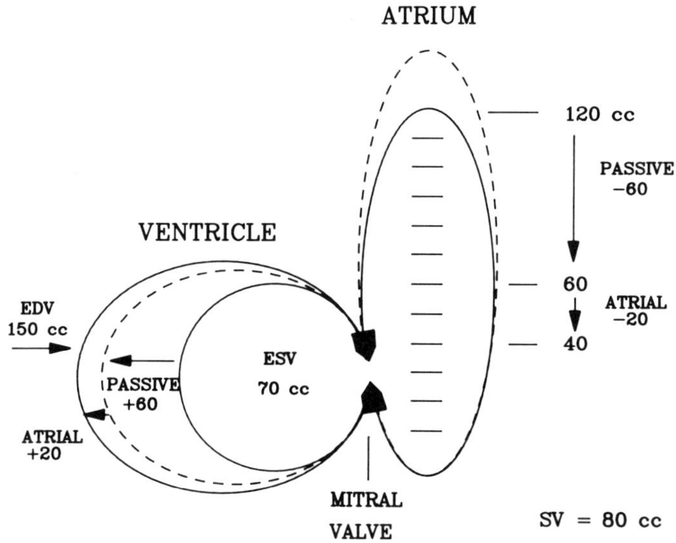

FIGURE 14. LV diastolic function, *reduced* loading (preload) conditions, *compliant* LV. This produces a mitral diastolic filling pattern as depicted in Figure 16A.

As with LV volumes, LV mass values are larger in normal men than in women (mean 148 g vs. 108 g, p <0.001) and these remain larger even after correcting for body surface area. Volume/mass ratios, however, are constant at end-diastole (0.80) and end-systole (0.26).[10]

III. SUMMARY

LV systolic function

A. Cardiac output (CO) and ejection fraction (EF)
   1. Echo methods
      a. M-mode Teicholz

$$V = \left[\frac{7.0}{2.4 + LVID}\right] LVID^3$$

$$SV = EDV - ESV$$

$$CO = SV \times HR$$

$$EF = \frac{EDV - ESV}{EDV} = \%$$

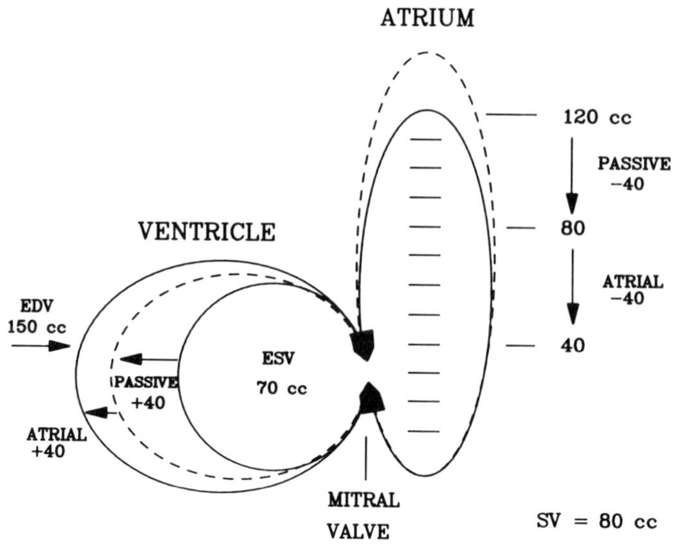

FIGURE 15. LV diastolic function, *reduced* loading (preload) conditions, *non-compliant* LV. This produces a mitral diastolic filling pattern as depicted in Figure 16B.

b. 2-D modified Simpson

Usually provided by computer programs in modern equipment.

2. Doppler method

$$CO\ (L/\min) = SV\ (\text{liters}) \times HR\ (BPM)$$

$$SV = TVI \times A\ (\text{AOR or LVOT}) = cm^3$$

$$TVI = \text{mean velocity} \times ET = cm$$

$$A = \pi\, r^2 = cm^2$$

$$SV = \frac{cm^3}{1000} = \text{liters}$$

$$CO = SV \times HR = l/\min$$

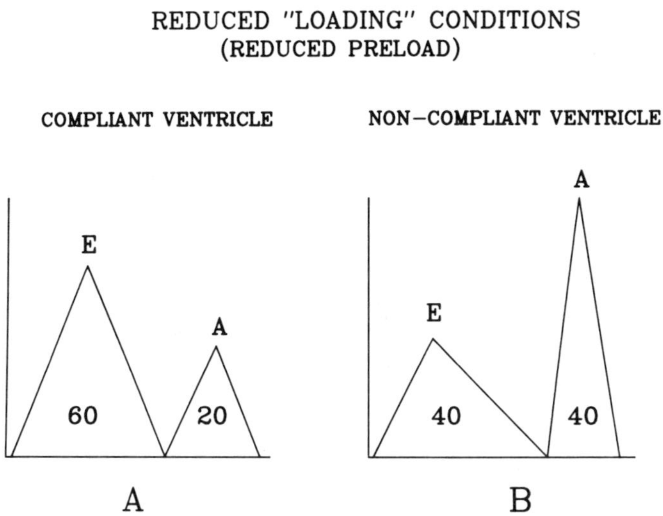

FIGURE 16. Mitral diastolic filling patterns under *reduced* loading (preload) conditions. Figure 16A is a compliant LV. Figure 16B is a noncompliant LV.

B. LV Mean ejection force (MEF)

$$\text{Force} = \text{mass} \times \text{acceleration}$$

$$M_{AT} = p \times TVI_{AT} \times CSA$$

$$p = 1.06\ g / cm^3$$

$$AA = \frac{PkV}{t}$$

$$MEF_{AT} = M_{AT} \times AA = \text{dynes}$$

Normal Values for MEF

MEF (K dynes)	29+5
MEF/BSA (K dynes/m^2)	17+3

LV DIASTOLIC FUNCTION

Typically, on the transmitral diastolic flow velocity profile (pulsed Doppler), impairment of LV filling produces a lower peak E, slowing in AT, greater slowing in DT, a higher peak A, and a decrease in the E:A ratio.

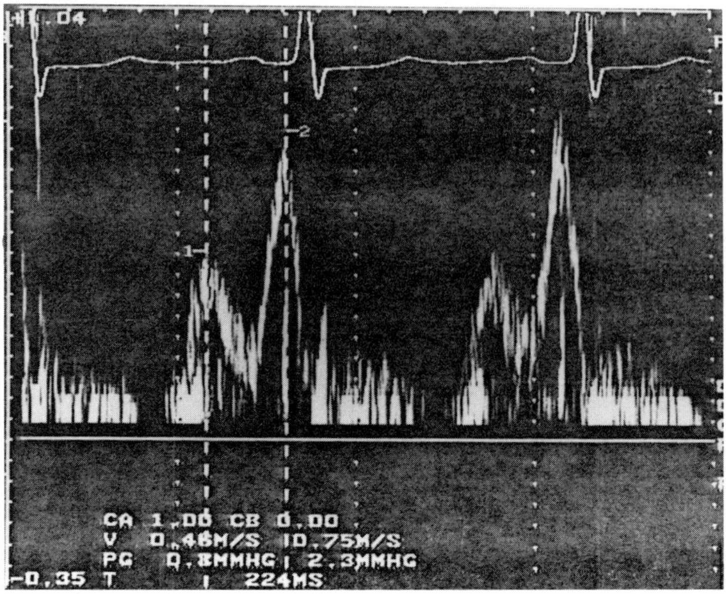

A

FIGURE 17. (A) Pulsed wave recording of transmitral diastolic flow velocity curve. Note early (E-wave) peak filling velocity (recorded at point "1") of 0.46 m/s. (B) Pulsed wave recording of transmitral diastolic flow velocity curve with computer-calculated mitral TVI of 0.17. Thus, the mitral peak filling rate normalized to mitral SV would be

$$\text{PFR} = \frac{\text{V (cm/s)}}{\text{TV Im (cm)}} = \frac{0.46}{0.17} = 2.71$$

An index of 2.71 clearly indicates impaired LV diastolic compliance in this patient.

The following values may be utilized:

Peak E (cm/s)	86 + 16
Peak A (cm/s)	56 + 13
Ratio E:A	1.6 + 0.5
AT (m/s)	73 + 10
DT (m/s)	199 + 32
E area/A area	2.7 + 0.51
A area/total area	0.28 + 0.04

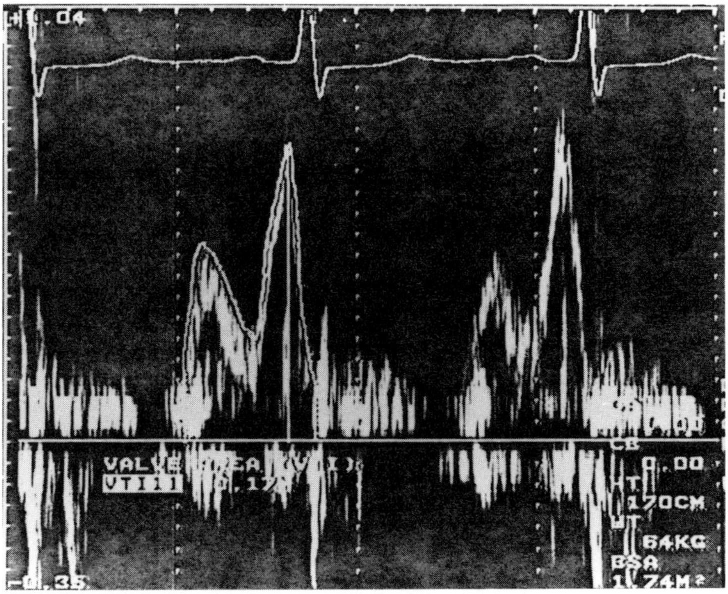

FIGURE 17B

Doppler *peak filling rate (PFR) normalized* to mitral SV (peak filling *index*):

$$\text{PFR}\,(\text{sv}/\text{s}) = \frac{\text{V}\,(\text{cm}/\text{s})}{\text{TV Im}\,(\text{cm})} = \text{index}$$

Normal *index* values are

$$\text{PFR} = 5.06 \pm 1.6$$

LV Mass (g)

Men	80–210
Women	75–150

REFERENCES

1. Teicholz, L. E., Kreulen, T., Herman, M. V., and Gorlin, R., Problems in echocardiographic volume determinations: echocardiographic-angiographic correlations in the presence or absence of asynergy, Am. J. Cardiol., 37, 7, 1976.
2. Falland, E. D., et al., Assessment of left ventricular ejection fraction by real-time, two dimensional echocardiography, Circulation, 60, 760, 1979.
3. Isaaz, K., et al., A new Doppler method of assessing left ventricular ejection force in chronic congestive heart failure, Am. J. Cardiol., 64, 81, 1989.
4. Lee, R. T., Plappert, M., and Sutton, M., Depressed left ventricular systolic ejection force in hypothyroidism, Am. J. Cardiol., 65, 526, 1990.
5. Rokey, R., Kuo, L. C., Zoghbi, W. A., Limacher, M. C., and Quinones, M. A., Determination of parameters of left ventricular diastolic filling with pulsed Doppler echocardiography, comparison with cineangiography, Circulation, 71, 543, 1985.
6. Nishiruma, R. A., et al., Assessment of diastolic function of the heart: background and current application of Doppler echocardiography, Parts 1 and 2, *Mayo Clin. Proc.*, 64, 181, 1989.
7. Appleton, C. P., et al., Demonstration of restrictive ventricular physiology by Doppler echocardiography, J. A*m*. C*oll.* C*ardiol.*, 11, 757, 1988.
8. deBruyne, B., et al., Doppler assessment of left ventricular diastolic filling during brief coronary occlusion, Am. Heart J., 117, 629, 1989.
9. Bowman, L. K., et al., Peak filling rate normalized to mitral stroke volume: a new Doppler echocardiographic filling index validated by radionuclide angiographic techniques, J. A*m*. C*oll.* C*ardiol.*, 12, 937, 1988.
10. Byrd, B. F., et al., Left ventricular mass and volume/mass ratio determined by two-dimensional echocardiography in normal adults, J. A*m*. C*oll.* C*ardiol.*, 6, 1021, 1985.

ADDITIONAL READING

Sabbah, H. N., et al., Non-invasive evaluation of left ventricular performance based on peak aortic blood acceleration measured with a continuous-wave Doppler velocity meter, Circulation, 74, 323, 1986.

Stork, T. V., et al., Non-invasive measurement of left ventricular filling pressures by means of transmitral pulsed Doppler ultrasound, Am. J. Cardiol., 64, 655, 1989.

Appleton, C. P., Hatle, L. K., and Popp, R. L., Relation of transmitral flow velocity patterns to left ventricular diastolic function: new insights from a combined hemodynamic and Doppler echocardiographic study, J. A*m*. C*oll.* C*ardiol.*, 12, 426, 1988.

Chapter 10

REGURGITANT FRACTIONS

I. DISCUSSION

In Chapters 4, 5 and 9, the methods for determining left ventricular (LV) and aortic root (AOR) stroke volume (SV) and flow (Q) were discussed as:

$$SV = TVI_a \times A_a$$

where TVI_a was the time velocity integral (TVI) (planimetered, or mean velocity × ejection time) of the LV-aortic systolic Doppler flow velocity profile and A_a was the area of the LV outflow tract (LVOT) or AOR.

As discussed partially in Chapter 6, the right ventricular (RV) and pulmonary artery (PA) SV and Q may be calculated using formulations similar to LV systolic flow. For the PA, the formulations are

$$SV = TVI_p \times A_p$$

where TVI_p is the TVI (planimetered, or mean velocity × ejection time) for the PA systolic velocity flow profile and A_p is the area of the pulmonary artery at the annulus. The A_p measurement is made on the 2-D short-axis view, in midsystole, at the base of the pulmonic cusps, for diameter, then utilize πr^2 for area calculation.

As noted before (Chapter 6) the walls of the PA in some patients may not be clearly identified and thus the diameter (d) of the PA cannot be accurately measured. In such instances, one may simply measure the excursion of the posterior (left) pulmonic valve cusp (usually easily visualized) and assume this is the radius (r) of the PA.[1]

In *aortic valvular insufficiency* (AI), the regurgitant fraction calculation is based on the comparison of pulmonic flow (QP) to aortic flow (QS). Since the heart rate for both chambers is identical, then SV may be substituted for flows.

Thus,

$$SV_a = \text{aortic stroke volume}$$

$$SV_p = \text{pulmonic stroke volume}$$

and, therefore, the regurgitant fraction in AI may be calculated as:

$$\frac{SV_a - SV_p}{SV_a} \times 100 = \%\ \text{regurgitant fraction}$$

An example might be an aortic SV of 120 cc (enhanced during systole by the AI produced abnormal LV filling during diastole) and a PA SV of 80 cc. Thus,

$$\frac{120-80}{120} = \frac{40}{120} = 33\%$$

In mitral valvular regurgitation, the aortic stroke volume (SV_a) is determined as described above and the LV stroke volume (LVSV) is determined by either M-mode or 2-D study (as described in Chapter 9). Thus, for mitral regurgitation the formula is

$$\frac{LVSV - SV_a}{LVSV} \times 100 = \% \text{ regurgitant fraction}$$

An example might be an LVSV of 120 cc and a SV_a of 80 cc. Thus,

$$\frac{120-80}{120} = \frac{40}{120} = 33\%$$

Regurgitant fractions exceeding 25% should be considered hemodynamically significant. Of interest would be the determinations of the acute and chronic effects of therapy (e.g., afterload reduction) on aortic and mitral valvular regurgitations utilizing the techniques described above.

II. SUMMARY

AI regurgitant fraction

SV_a = aortic stroke volume (Doppler)
SV_p = pulmonic stroke volume (Doppler)

$$\frac{SV_a - SV_p}{SV_a} \times 100 = \% \text{ AI regurgitant fraction}$$

MR regurgitant fraction

ASV = aortic stroke volume (Doppler)
LVSV = left ventricular stroke volume (2-D Simpson or M-mode Teicholz)

$$\frac{LVSV - ASV}{LVSV} \times 100 = \% \text{ MR regurgitant fraction}$$

REFERENCES

1. **Giroud, J., Pickoff, A. S., and Ferrer, P. L.,** Pulsed Doppler echocardiographic quantification of left-to-right shunts in children with isolated ventricular septal defect, in *Cardiac Doppler Diagnosis,* Spencer, M. P., Ed., Martinius Nijhoff, The Hague, 227,

ADDITIONAL READING

Rokey, R., et al., Determination of regurgitant fraction in isolated mitral or aortic regurgitation by pulsed Doppler two-dimensional echocardiography, *J. Am. Coll. Cardiol.,* 7, 1273, 1986.

Miyatake, K., et al., Semiquantitative grading of severity of mitral regurgitation by real-time two-dimensional Doppler flow imaging technique, *J. Am. Coll. Cardiol.,* 7, 82, 1986.

Chapter 11

INTRACARDIAC SHUNTS AND PULMONARY-TO-SYSTEMIC FLOW RATIOS (QP:QS)

I. DISCUSSION

The basic information needed and formulations utilized in calculations of shunt ratios have been already provided in Chapters 4 to 6, 9, and 10. Recall:

$$F = V \times A$$

where F(Q) is flow, V is velocity, and A is area. For the relevant calculations of pulmonary and systemic flows then one needs the peak pulmonary artery flow velocity curve [parasternal short axis, pulsed, or best CW), the peak aortic flow velocity curve (apical or parasternal windows, best continuous wave (CW)], the pulmonary artery (PA) dimensions (parasternal short axis), and the left ventricular (LV) outflow tract, aortic valve (Ao) dimensions (parasternal long-axis view).

Thus, pulmonary-to-aortic flow ratio can be estimated as:

$$\frac{F_p}{F_a} = \frac{\text{PA V max} \times (\text{PAd})^2}{\text{Ao V max} \times (\text{Aod})^2} = \text{QP:QS ratio}$$

where F_p is pulmonary flow, F_a is aortic flow, PA Vmax is maximum flow velocity in the PA, Ao Vmax is the maximum aortic flow, PAd is the PA diameter and Aod is the aortic valve diameter. (Note that either diameters or radii may be utilized in these calculations since it is a *ratio* which is being calculated. Likewise, π need not be utilized.)

Since there are some variations in the ejection times of the right heart as compared to the left heart, a more precise calculation would be

$$\frac{F_p}{F_a} = \frac{\text{TVI}_p \times (\text{PAd})^2}{\text{TVI}_a \times (\text{Aod})^2}$$

where TVI_p and TVI_a are the time velocity integrals (planimetered or mean velocity × ejection time) of the pulmonary artery and aortic outflow, respectively.

Utilizing the above, shunt ratios for atrial septal defect (QP:QS) and for ventricular septal defect (QP:QS) may be estimated.

Assume, with a shunt, the TVI_p is 28, the TVI_a is 24, the PAd is 2.2, and the Aod is 2.0. Therefore,

$$\frac{28}{24} \times \frac{(2.2)^2}{(2)^2} = \frac{28}{24} \times \frac{4.84}{4} = \frac{135.52}{96} = 1.4$$

Thus, the QP:QS or shunt ratio is 1.4:1.

II. SUMMARY

Shunts for ASD and VSD are estimated by the QP:QS ratio as:

$$\frac{QP}{QS} = \frac{TVI_p \times (PAd)^2}{TVI_s \times (Aod)^2} = \text{ratio}$$

ADDITIONAL READING

Sanders, S. P., Yeager, S., and Williams, R. G., Measurement of systemic and pulmonary blood flow and QP:QS ratio using Doppler and two-dimensional echocardiography, *Am. J. Cardiol.*, 51, 952, 1983.

Valdes-Cruz, L. M., et al., A pulsed Doppler echocardiographic method for calculating pulmonary and systemic blood flow in atrial level shunts: validation studies in animals and initial human experience, *Circulation*, 69, 80, 1984.

Chapter 12

PERICARDIAL DISEASE

I. PERICARDIAL EFFUSION AND CARDIAC TAMPONADE

Fairly reliable predictors of the presence of cardiac tamponade in pericardial effusions have been established by M-mode and 2-D echocardiography, particularly early diastolic collapse of the right ventricle and late diastolic collapse of the right atrium. Less attention has been given to Doppler-derived data in tamponade, however. Initial studies in this disorder revealed increased respiratory variation in transvalvular flow velocities produced by pulsed-wave Doppler examination.[1-3] A more recent study[4] confirmed prior data and provided Doppler information in cardiac tamponade that can be easily obtained, analyzed, and applied clinically. This study addressed primarily pulsed-wave Doppler-derived diastolic transmitral and transtricuspid valve profiles. The mitral valve E-wave (cm/s) and mitral time velocity integral (TVI, cm) were similar in normal subjects and in patients with pericardial effusions but without tamponade, throughout the respiratory cycle. In patients with tamponade, however, the mitral E-wave and TVI were significantly lower (each essentially exceeding 25%) during inspiration when compared to expiration. As would be expected, tricuspid E-wave and TVI were highest during inspiration in normal subjects and patients with pericardial effusions (with or without tamponade), reflecting the anticipated augmentation of filling of the right heart during *inspiration*. Compared to others, in patients with tamponade, during *expiration* there was a marked decrease in the tricuspid E-wave and TVI. This produced wide swings during the respiratory cycle between inspiration and expiration in the tamponade group. Comparing the *tricuspid E-wave* (cm/s) and *TVI* (cm) *variations from expiration to inspiration* revealed essentially the following changes: (l) normal subjects and patients with effusion but no tamponade, a variation of less than 15% and (2) patients with tamponade, a variation of more than 40%.

Figure 1 displays the normal transmitral diastolic flow profile during expiration and inspiration.

Figure 2 displays the abnormal respiratory variation in the mitral diastolic flow profiles encountered in patients with tamponade.

Figure 3 displays the normal transtricuspid diastolic flow profile during inspiration and expiration.

Figures 4A and B display the abnormal respiratory variation in tricuspid diastolic flow profiles encountered in patients with tamponade.

These transvalvular flow velocity variations with respiration are reliable with tamponade even in the absence of imaging display of right ventricular or right atrial collapse.

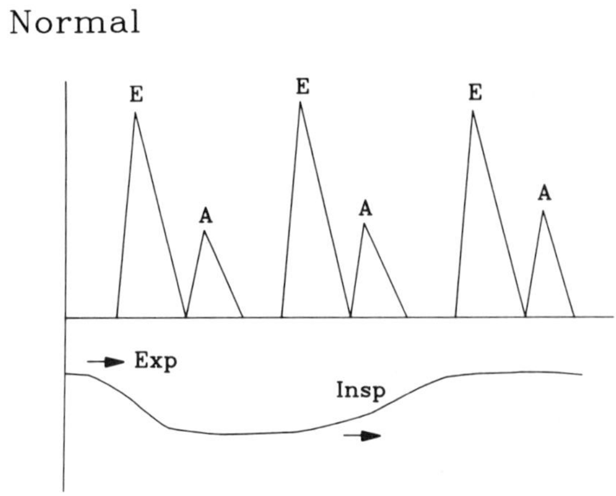

FIGURE 1. Diagrammatic representation of a transmitral diastolic flow profile from a normal subject. Note very minimal variation in the flow patterns from expiration to inspiration (adapted from Bristow et al.[4]).

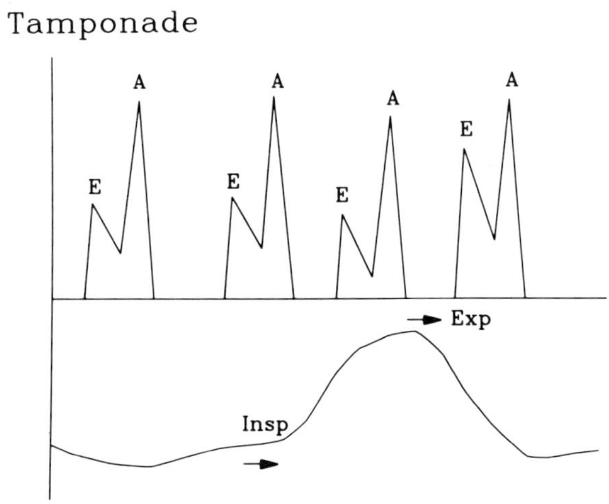

FIGURE 2. Diagrammatic representation of transmitral diastolic flow profiles from a patient with tamponade. Note the decrease in the E wave during the first beat of inspiration and the increase in the E wave during the first beat of expiration (adapted from Bristow et al.[4]).

II. CONSTRICTIVE PERICARDITIS

In constrictive pericarditis (CP) from whatever cause, the rigid "ungiving" pericardium impedes filling of the enclosed cardiac chambers. As such, most

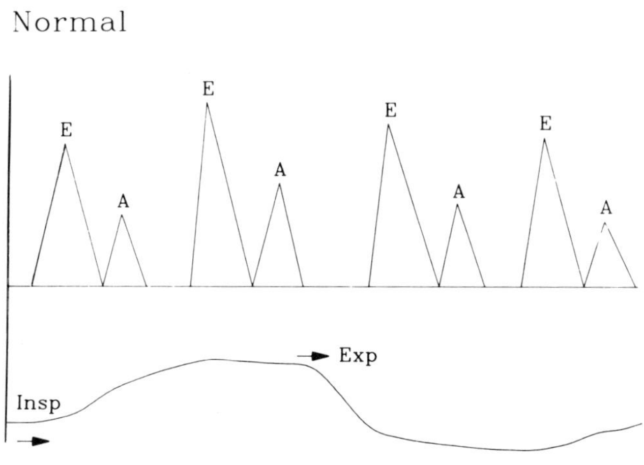

FIGURE 3. Diagrammatic representation of the transtricuspid diastolic flow profile from a normal subject. Note the normal increase in the E-wave during inspiration (anticipated normal increase in RV filling during inspiration). During expiration there is a minimal decrease in the E-wave amplitude (adapted from Bristow et al.[4]).

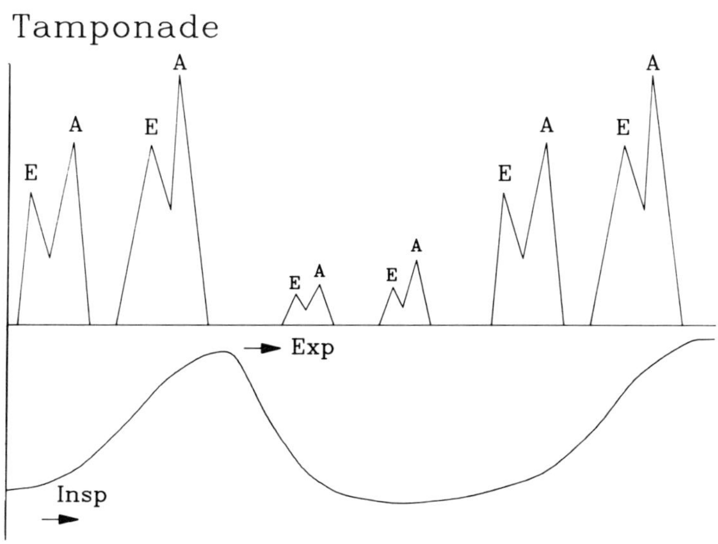

FIGURE 4A. Diagrammatic representation of transtricuspid diastolic flow profile from a patient with tamponade. Note the increase in flow velocities during inspiration. On the first two beats of expiration, note the almost total loss of tricuspid flow velocity (adapted from Bristow et al.[4]).

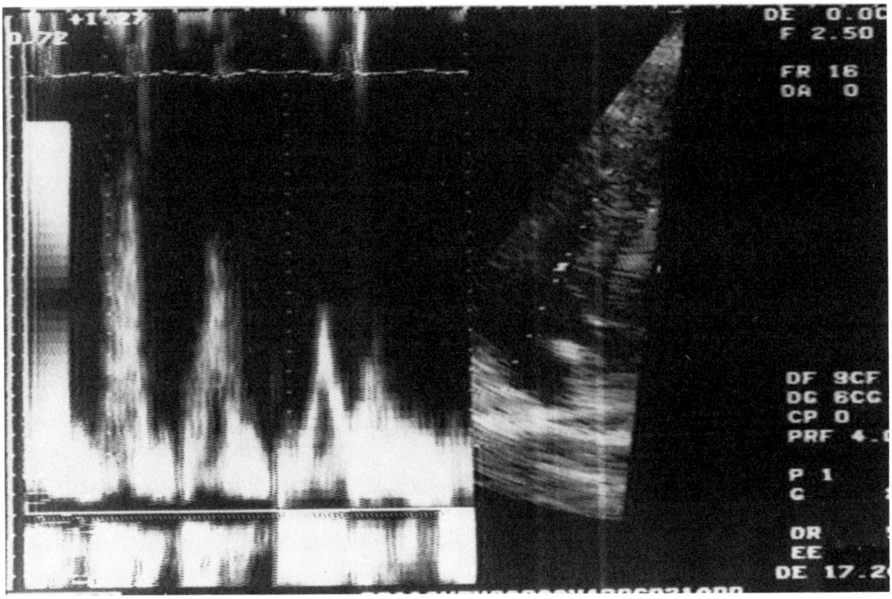

FIGURE 4B. Actual recording (PW) of the transtricuspid diastolic velocity flow profile from a patient with pericardial effusion and tamporade. Note the marked decrease in velocities that occur from inspiration (to the left) to expiration (to the right). Insert 2D view shows the Doppler PW sample volume placed in the RV below the tricuspid valve.

of ventricular filling takes place during the first one third of diastole. This results in the well-known diastolic "dip and plateau" or "square-root sign" on the hemodynamic profile. Exaggerated respiratory variations in LV and RV filling patterns are expected. Thus, Doppler findings helpful in the diagnosis of CP are (l) excessive (>25%) decrease in mitral diastolic (E) velocity during *inspiration,* (2) excessive (>25%) decrease in tricuspid diastolic (E) velocity during *expiration,* (3) prominent mitral and tricuspid diastolic "E" in comparison to "A", because of the predominance of early diastolic filling in CP (Figure 5), and (4) a shortened mitral and tricuspid pressure half-time reflecting the "dip and plateau" ventricular pressure configuration with abrupt cessation of ventricular filling. Normal pressure half-times range from 20 to 60 m/s.

Differentiation between CP and restrictive cardiomyopathy may be difficult. Criteria to assist in this differentiation have recently been published.[5]

III. SUMMARY

Pericardial tamponade

Compare E and TVI during inspiration to that during expiration:

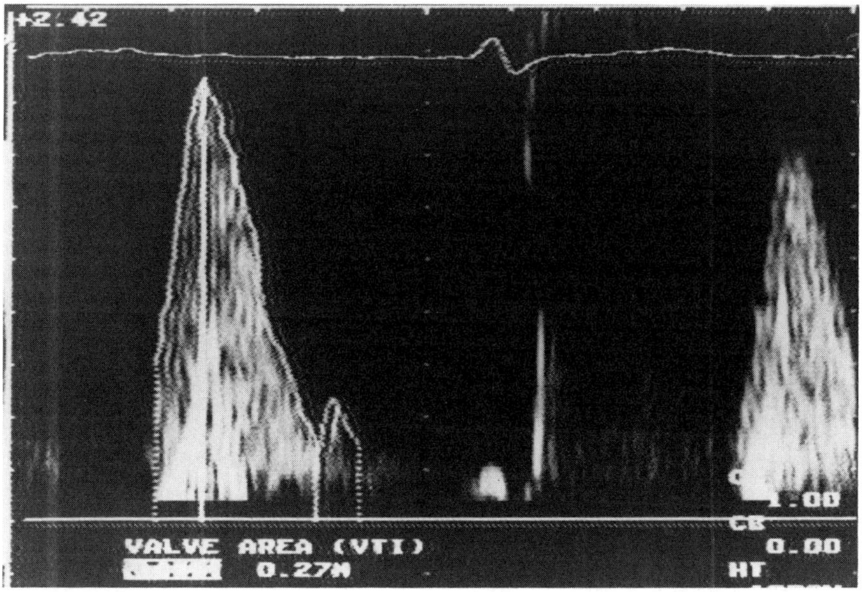

FIGURE 5. Transmitral CW flow profile from a patient with constrictive pericarditis. Note the abrupt "total" filling in early diastole.

1. Mitral is lower (>25%) during inspiration.
2. Tricuspid variation is higher in tamponade (>40%) than in its absence (<15%).

Constrictive pericarditis

1. Excessive (>25%) decreased mitral E during inspiration.
2. Excessive (>25%) decreased tricuspid E during expiration.
3. Prominent mitral and tricuspid E compared to A.
4. Shortened mitral and tricuspid pressure half-times. Normal is 20 to 60 m/s.

REFERENCES

1. **Pandian, N. G., Wang, S. S., McInerney, K., Caldeira, M., Konstam, M. A., Isner, J. M., and Salem, D. N.,** Doppler echocardiography in cardiac tamponade: abnormalities in tricuspid and mitral flow response to respiration in experimental and clinical tamponade, *J. Am. Coll. Cardiol.,* 5(abstr.), 485, 1985.
2. **Leeman, D. E., Levine, M. J., and Come, P. C.,** Doppler echocardiography in cardiac tamponade: exaggerated respiratory variation in transvalvular blood flow velocity integrals, *J. Am. Coll. Cardiol.,* 11, 572, 1988.
3. **Appleton, C. P., Hatle, L. K., and Popp, R. L.,** Cardiac tamponade and pericardial effusion: respiratory variation in transvalvular flow velocities studied by Doppler echocardiography, *J. Am. Coll. Cardiol.,* 11, 1020, 1988.
4. **Burstow, D., Oh, J., Bailey, K. R., Seward, J. B., and Tajik, A. J.,** Cardiac tamponade: characteristic Doppler observations, *Mayo Clin. Proc.,* 64, 313, 1989.
5. **Hatle, L. K., Appleton, C. P., and Popp, R. L.,** Differentiation of constrictive pericarditis and restrictive cardiomyopathy by Doppler echocardiography, *Circulation,* 79, 357, 1989.

ADDITIONAL READING

Bibra, H. V., et al., Diagnosis of constrictive pericarditis by pulsed Doppler echocardiography of the hepatic vein, *Am. J. Cardiol.,* 63, 483, 1989.

Himelman, R. B., Kircher, B., Rockey, D. C., and Schiller, N. B., Inferior vena cava plethora with blunted respiratory response: a sensitive echocardiographic sign of cardiac tamponade, *J. Am. Coll. Cardiol.,* 12, 1470, 1988.

ABBREVIATIONS

AA	— Aortic valve annulus
AI or AR	— Aortic insufficiency or regurgitation
AOR or AR	— Aortic root
AOV or AV	— Aortic valve
APM	— Anterior papillary muscle
AS	— Aortic stenosis
ASD	— Atrial septal defect
AVA	— Aortic valve area
BP	— Blood pressure
cm/s	— Centimeters per second
CO	— Cardiac output
CW	— Continuous wave
ET	— Ejection time
F	— Flow
G	— Gradient
HR	— Heart rate
IAS	— Interatrial septum
IVC	— Inferior vena cava
IVS	— Interventricular septum
LA	— Left atrium
LAX	— Long axis
LCC	— Left coronary cusp of aortic valve
LV	— Left ventricle
LVOT	— Left ventricular outflow tract
MB	— Moderator band
ms	— Milliseconds
M/s or m/s	— Meters per second
mmHg	— Millimeters of mercury
MR	— Mitral regurgitation
MS	— Mitral stenosis
MVA	— Mitral valve area
NCC	— Noncoronary cusp of aortic valve
PA	— Pulmonary artery
PAA	— Pulmonary artery annulus
PAP	— Pulmonary artery pressure
PCW	— Pulmonary capillary wedge pressure
PD	— Pulsed Doppler
PDA	— Patent ductus arteriosus
P1/2t	— Pressure half-time
PI or PR	— Pulmonic valve insufficiency or regurgitation

PM	— Papillary muscle
PPM	— Posterior papillary muscle
PRF	— Pulse repetition frequency
PS	— Pulmonic valve stenosis
PV-A or APV	— Anterior cusp of the pulmonic valve
PV	— Pulmonic valve
PV-L, PV-P, LPV or PPV	— Left or posterior cusp of pulmonic valve
Q	— Flow
RA	— Right atrium
RCC	— Right coronary cusp of aortic valve
RV	— Right ventricle
SAX	— Short axis
s	— Seconds
SVC	— Superior vena cava
TR or TI	— Tricuspid valve regurgitation or insufficiency
TS	— Tricuspid stenosis
TV	— Tricuspid valve
TV-A or ATV	— Anterior tricuspid valve leaflet
TVI	— Time velocity integral
TV-P or PTV	— Posterior tricuspid valve leaflet
TV-S or STV	— Septal tricuspid valve leaflet
V, Vel	— Velocity (in context)
VA	— Ventricular aneurysm
Vmax	— Maximum velocity
V, Vol	— Volume (in context)
VSD	— Ventricular septal defect

APPENDIX A

TECHNICAL TIPS

These technical tips are presented to reinforce some of the basic principles in performing a Doppler echocardiographic exam.

First, a few general Doppler tips which can be applied to most situations when obtaining spectral flow patterns for qualitative and quantitative purposes follow.

The importance of taking great care and time to align the ultrasonic beam parallel to the appropriate jet being interrogated cannot be overemphasized, especially in quantitative Doppler echocardiography.

Using the image-guide color-coded pulsed-Doppler technique, the sample volume can be placed in the area of brightest color and if aliasing is present, continuous wave Doppler can be used to obtain higher velocities.

Multiple transducer positions or acoustic windows obtained by movement in small increments and various angulation should be used to find the highest velocity (brightest color or aliasing). This will also help to find maximal color jet size for regurgitant jets.

Other important tips are the use of audio signals to assist in finding higher velocities and positioning the patient in a left lateral position (for left intercostal transducer placement) and a right lateral position (for right intercostal transducer placement).

The spectral pattern obtained should be well defined and several samples taken and averaged (quantitatively) to eliminate small sources of error. There should be three to five samples for a normal sinus rhythm and up to 10 samples for atrial fibrillation. Other potential sources of error which may contribute to inaccurate results are various arrhythmias, heart rate (which can change diastolic filling time and cardiac output), and patient movement and respiration.

Second, these tips are presented in relation to the specific valves, giving some information which might be valuable in obtaining a better exam.

Transmitral flow is usually best obtained with the various apical views and left parasternal views. Here, the left lateral position can greatly enhance the exam and allow a higher PRF to be used.

Interrogate the left ventricle from the apex and move the sample volume down to and through the mitral valve (being careful to avoid a false positive diagnosis of mitral regurgitation when the sample volume is <1 cm from the mitral valve). A posterosuperior direction of the ultrasonic beam will often aid in maximizing the transmitral pattern. Color Doppler is very useful for the initial search of the MR jet (as well as other regurgitant jets) and continuous wave Doppler will usually be necessary for the higher velocities associated with pathological jets.

Blood flow through the aortic valve is usually best obtained in the 3 or 5 chamber apical views. In addition, aortic flow can be obtained in the suprasternal and high right parasternal (with right lateral positioning) views. Interrogating the valve >1 cm above and below the valve will aid in avoiding artifacts.

Transtricuspid flow is obtained with the apical, left parasternal (short and long axis) and subcostal views. Interrogating the tricuspid valve in the same manner as the mitral valve will usually give adequate results. One important point is the respiratory variation seen with transtricuspid spectral patterns. With superficial respiration this problem however can be minimized.

Pulmonic flow is best obtained in the left parasternal short axis and in a small subset of patients the subcostal view is useful. In the parasternal view an inferior tilt of the transducer can often aid in finding the maximum velocity. Also, two to four intercostal spaces should be attempted in this view. Interrogating the valve above and below in a manner similar to the aortic valve is necessary.

The left to right flow seen in atrial septal defects can be obtained in the left parasternal (short or long axis) and the subcostal view. Interrogating the right side of the interatrial septum along its length with pulsed wave (color-coded) Doppler can be used to analyze the flow from an ASD, which will usually have velocities lower than the Nyquist limit. There is usually an increase in the tricuspid flow which can aid in the diagnosis of an ASD.

The left to right flow seen in ventricular septal defects can be obtained in the apical, left parasternal, or subcostal views. Interrogating the right side of the ventricular septum along its length in the same manner as the atrial septum (for an ASD) can be used, but continuous wave Doppler will often be needed to quantitate the higher velocities seen with ventricular septal defects.

APPENDIX B

Accompanying are cardiac Doppler "worksheets" which we have found to be of value. Data from the completion of these forms can be transferred easily into a final dictated report.

Blank worksheet forms are noted, followed by completed worksheet forms illustrating the following: (1) moderately severe AS and AI, (2) moderate to advanced AI, and (3) moderate MS.

TULANE UNIVERSITY MEDICAL CENTER CARDIAC DOPPLER WORKSHEET	NAME:		
	PT. #:		
	AGE:		SEX:
	HT.(in.)	WT.(lbs.)	BSA(m^2)

AORTIC VALVE

Systole

peak velocity______m/s (<1.7 m/s)
mean velocity______m/s
peak gradient______mmHg
mean gradient______(>50 mmHg, severe)
V_1V_2
tP/tQ
AVA(cont. eqn.)______cm^2 (>2.2 cm^2, "insignificant")

LVOT: area______cm^2 vel______m/s
AO: area______cm^2 vel______m/s

Diastole (AI)

peak velocity______m/s
mean velocity______m/s
peak gradient______mmHg
mean gradient______mmHg

AIJA/LVOTA______%(sax)
AIJH/LVOTH______%(lax)
timing AI jet ______ms
$P^1/_2$ time ______ms (500 ms)

Evaluation: ______________________ ______________________

______________________ ______________________

MITRAL VALVE

Diastole

peak velocity______m/s (<1.3 m/s)
mean velocity______m/s
peak gradient______mmHg
mean gradient______mmHg
$P^1/_2$ ______ms
MVA(cont. eqn.)______cm^2 (4–6 cm^2)
(planimeter)______cm^2 (4–6 cm^2)
($P^1/_2$ time) ______cm^2 (>2.2 cm^2)
E/A ratio ______(1.1–2.1)
pk v./mean v. ______
pk v. normalized to mitral stroke volume ______(5.06 ± 1.6)

Evaluation: ______________________

____

Systole (MR)

peak velocity______m/s (>1.5 m/s,PW)
mean velocity______m/s
peak gradient______mmHg
mean gradient______mmHg
MRJA/LAA%______(>20%, sign.)
timing MR jet______ms (N < 100 ms)

Evaluation: ______________________

____

TULANE UNIVERSITY MEDICAL CENTER CARDIAC DOPPLER WORKSHEET

NAME:
PT. #:
AGE: SEX:
HT.(in.) WT.(lbs.) BSA(m^2)

PULMONIC VALVE

Systole

peak velocity______m/s(<0.9 m/s)
mean velocity______m/s
peak gradient______mmHg
mean gradient______mmHg

Evaluation:__________________________
____

Diastole (PI)

peak velocity______m/s
mean velocity______m/s
peak gradient______mmHg
mean gradient______mmHg
$P_{1/2}$ time ______ms
timing ______ms

Evaluation:__________________________
____

TRICUSPID VALVE

Diastole

peak velocity______m/s(<0.8 m/s)
mean velocity______m/s
peak gradient______mmHg
mean gradient______mmHg

Evaluation:__________________________
____

Systole (TR)

peak velocity______m/s
mean velocity______m/s
peak gradient______mmHg
mean gradient______mmHg
TRJA/RAA%______%
timing ______ms

Evaluation:__________________________
____

PRESSURES (mmHg)

Blood Pressure (cuff)	systolic______	diastolic[1]______
		diastolic[2]______
Left Ventricle	systolic______	end diastolic ______(A)
Right Ventricle	systolic______(TR)	
Pulmonary Artery	systolic______	mean

IVC diameter__________(N < 1.5 cm, dilated > 2.0 cm)
respiratory compression__________%(N > 50%)

FINAL REPORT DICTATED FROM COMPLETED WORKSHEET EXAMPLE #1

Multiple cardiac Doppler flow studies were obtained in the standard areas. The study was assisted with color flow mapping. An abnormal aortic valve was noted on the 2-D echo and in this context there was evidence of moderate aortic valvular insufficiency. There was also evidence of moderate to severe aortic stenosis. The peak systolic gradient across the aortic valve was 59 mmHg and the mean gradient was 34 mmHg. The calculated aortic valve area (continuity equation) was 1.02 cm^2 after being "corrected" for the moderately severe aortic valvular insufficiency. No abnormalities were detected in association with the mitral, pulmonic, or tricuspid valves. There was no evidence of any significant pulmonary hypertension.

TULANE UNIVERSITY MEDICAL CENTER CARDIAC DOPPLER WORKSHEET

NAME:
PT. #:
AGE: SEX:
HT.(in.) WT.(lbs.) $BSA(m^2)$

AORTIC VALVE

Systole

peak velocity *3.84* m/s (<1.7 m/s)
mean velocity *2.91* m/s
peak gradient *59.0* mmHg
mean gradient *33.9* (>50 mmHg, severe)
V_1V_2 *0.33* (n = 1)
tP/tQ ______ (n < 40%)
AVA(cont. eqn.) *1.02* cm^2 (>2.2 cm^2, "insignificant")

LVOT: area *310* cm^2 vel *0.95* m/s
AO: area ______ cm^2 vel *3.84* m/s

Evaluation: *Moderate to severe aortic stenosis with correction for aortic insufficiency*

Diastole (AI)

peak velocity *4.08* m/s
mean velocity *3.52* m/s
peak gradient *66.6* mmHg
mean gradient *49.6* mmHg
End diastolic velocity *3.46* m/s
End diastolic gradient *47.9* mmHg
AIJA/LVOTA *30* %(sax)
AIJH/LVOTH *60* %(lax)
timing AI jet *400* ms
$P^{1/2}$ time *256* ms (500 ms)

Evaluation: *Moderate aortic insufficiency*

MITRAL VALVE

Diastole

peak velocity *1.03* m/s (<1.3 m/s)
mean velocity *0.44* m/s
peak gradient *4.24* mmHg
mean gradient *0.77* mmHg
$P^{1/2}$ *31* ms
MVA(cont. eqn.) — cm^2 (4–6 cm^2)
(planimeter) — cm^2 (4–6 cm^2)
($P^{1/2}$ time) *7.10* cm^2 (>2.2 cm^2)
E/A ratio *2.0* (1.1–2.1)
pk v./mean v. *2.34*
pk v. normalized to mitral stroke volume *5.73* (5.06 ± 1.6)

Evaluation: *Within normal limits*

Systole (MR)

peak velocity ______ m/s (>1.5 m/s,PW)
mean velocity ______ m/s
peak gradient ______ mmHg
mean gradient ______ mmHg
MRJA/LAA% ______ (>20%, sign.)
timing MR jet ______ ms (N < 100 ms)

Evaluation: *MR not detected*

FINAL REPORT DICTATED FROM COMPLETED WORK SHEET EXAMPLE #2

Multiple cardiac Doppler flow studies were obtained in the standard areas. The study was assisted by color flow mapping. An abnormal aortic root and aortic valve were noted on the 2D echo and in this context there was evidence of moderate to severe aortic valvular insufficiency. There was no significant aortic stenosis. No abnormalities were detected in association with the mitral, tricuspid, or pulmonic valves. There was no significant pulmonary hypertension.

TULANE UNIVERSITY MEDICAL CENTER CARDIAC DOPPLER WORKSHEET

NAME:
PT. #:
AGE: SEX:
HT.(in.) WT.(lbs.) BSA(m^2)

AORTIC VALVE

Systole

peak velocity *1.38* m/s (<1.7 m/s)
mean velocity *1.06* m/s
peak gradient *7.6* mmHg
mean gradient *4.6* (>50 mmHg, severe)
V_1V_2 *0.98* (n = 1)
tP/tQ ______ (n < 40%)
AVA(cont. eqn.) *3.65* cm^2 (>2.2 cm^2, "insignificant")

LVOT: area *3.73* cm^2 vel *1.35* m/s
AO: area ______ cm^2 vel *1.38* m/s

Evaluation: *Within normal limits*

Diastole (AI)

peak velocity *4.23* m/s
mean velocity *3.31* m/s
peak gradient *71.6* mmHg
mean gradient *43.3* mmHg
End diastolic velocity *2.37* m/s
End diastolic gradient *22.5* mmHg
AIJA/LVOTA *40* %(sax)
AIJH/LVOTH *70* %(lax)
timing AI jet *490* ms
P½ time *244* ms (500 ms)

Evaluation: *Moderate to severe aortic* insufficiency

MITRAL VALVE

Diastole

peak velocity *0.96* m/s (<1.3 m/s)
mean velocity *0.41* m/s
peak gradient *3.7* mmHg
mean gradient *0.7* mmHg
P½ *28* ms
MVA(cont. eqn.) — cm^2 (4–6 cm^2)
(planimeter) — cm^2 (4–6 cm^2)
(P½ time) *7.86* cm^2 (>2.2 cm^2)
E/A ratio *1.7* (1.1–2.1)
pk v./mean v. *2.34*
pk v. normalized to mitral stroke volume *5.33* (5.06 ± 1.6)

Evaluation: *Within normal limits*

Systole (MR)

peak velocity ______ m/s (>1.5 m/s,PW)
mean velocity ______ m/s
peak gradient ______ mmHg
mean gradient ______ mmHg
MRJA/LAA% ______ (>20%, sign.)
timing MR jet ______ ms (N < 100 ms)

Evaluation: *MR not detected*

FINAL REPORT DICTATED FROM COMPLETED WORKSHEET EXAMPLE #3

Multiple cardiac Doppler flow studies were obtained in the standard areas. The study was assisted by color flow mapping. No abnormalities were detected in association with the aortic valve. An abnormal mitral valve was noted on the 2-D echo and in this context there was evidence of moderate mitral stenosis. The peak diastolic gradient was 18 mmHg. The pressure half-time was 344 m/s. The mitral valve area calculated by the pressure half-time method was 0.64 cm^2. The planimetered mitral valve orifice was 0.72 cm^2. There was no evidence of any significant mitral regurgitation. There was evidence of mild to moderate pulmonary hypertension with a systolic pressure of 38 mmHg (calculated from the tricuspid regurgitant jet) and a mean pressure of 28 mmHg (calculated from 80-1/2 acceleration time). There was evidence of mild to moderate pulmonic valvular insufficiency and mild to moderate tricuspid regurgitation.

TULANE UNIVERSITY MEDICAL CENTER CARDIAC DOPPLER WORKSHEET

NAME:
PT. #:
AGE: SEX:
HT.(in.) WT.(lbs.) BSA(m^2)

AORTIC VALVE

Systole

peak velocity *1.21* m/s (<1.7 m/s)
mean velocity *0.92* m/s
peak gradient *6.66* mmHg
mean gradient *4.03* (>50 mmHg, severe)
V_1V_2 *0.96* (n = 1)
tP/tQ ______(n < 40%)
AVA(cont. eqn.) *3.57* cm^2 (>2.2 cm^2, "insignificant")

LVOT: area *3.66* cm^2 vel *1.18* m/s
AO: area ______ cm^2 vel *1.21* m/s

Evaluation: *Within normal limits*

Diastole (AI)

peak velocity ______ m/s
mean velocity ______ m/s
peak gradient ______ mmHg
mean gradient ______ mmHg
End diastolic velocity ______ m/s
End diastolic gradient ______ mmHg
AIJA/LVOTA ______ %(sax)
AIJH/LVOTH ______ %(lax)
timing AI jet ______ ms
P½ time ______ ms (500 ms)

Evaluation: *AI not detected*

MITRAL VALVE

Diastole

peak velocity *2.14* m/s (<1.3 m/s)
mean velocity *1.60* m/s
peak gradient *18.32* mmHg
mean gradient *10.24* mmHg
P½ *344* ms
MVA(cont. eqn.) ______ cm^2 (4–6 cm^2)
(planimeter) 0.72 cm^2 (4–6 cm^2)
(P½ time) *0.64* cm^2 (>2.2 cm^2)
E/A ratio *1.13* (1.1–2.1)
pk v./mean v. *1.34*
pk v. normalized to mitral stroke volume *1.8* (5.06 ± 1.6)

Evaluation: *Moderate mitral stenosis*

Systole (MR)

peak velocity ______ m/s (>1.5 m/s,PW)
mean velocity ______ m/s
peak gradient ______ mmHg
mean gradient ______ mmHg
MRJA/LAA% ______ (>20%, sign.)
timing MR jet ______ ms (N < 100 ms)

Evaluation: *MR not detected*

APPENDIX C

NORMAL VALUES

I. Pressures (mmHg)

Left Ventricle (LV)	
Peak systolic/end diastolic (LVEDP)	100–140/3–12
Right Ventricle (RV)	
Peak systolic/end diastolic (RVEDP)	15–30/1–8
Left Atrium	
Mean diastolic	1–10
Right Atrium	
Mean diastolic	0–5
Systemic Arterial	
Peak systolic/end diastolic	100–140/60–90
Pulmonary artery	
Peak systolic/end diastolic	15–30/5–12
Mean	10–18

II. Left ventricular function

A. Systolic

Stroke volume (cc/beat)	70–140
Stroke index (cc/beat/m2)	30–60
Cardiac output (l/min)	4–7
Cardiac index (l/min/m2)	2.5–4.5
Acceleration time	
Peak velocity (cm/s)	108 ± 7
Mean acceleration (cm/s/s)	1209 ± 28
Accelerated blood mass (g)	25 ± 6
Mean ejection force (K dynes)	29 ± 5
Ejection fraction (o/o)	55–75

B. Diastolic	Tricuspid	Mitral
Peak E (cm/s)	57 ± 8	86 ± 16
Peak A (cm/s)	39 ± 6	56 ± 13
Ratio E:A	1.5 ± 0.3	1.6 ± 0.5
Acceleration time (m/s)	83 ± 14	73 ± 10
Deceleration time (m/s)	225 ± 28	199 ± 32
E area/A area		2.7 ± 0.51
A area/total area		0.28 ± 0.04
Peak filling rate index (s)		5.06 ± 1.6

III. **Flow velocities (m/s)**

Aortic valve	1.0 – 1.7
Mitral valve	0.6 – 1.3
Pulmonic valve	0.4 – 1.0
Tricuspid valve	0.3 – 0.8

IV. **Valve areas (cm^2)**

Aortic	2.6 – 3.6
Mitral	4 – 7
Pulmonic	3.5 – 4.5
Tricuspid	5 – 8

V. **Pressure Half-Times (m/s)**

Mitral	20 – 60

VI. **Inferior vena cava parameters**

Diameter (expiration) (mm)	9 – 15
Collapsibility (inspiration) (0/0)	50 – 100

VII. **Prosthetic valves** (see Summary of Chapter 8)

VIII. **Left ventricular mass (Gm)**

Men	80 – 210
Women	75 – 150

VALUES FOR COMMON ABNORMALITIES

I. Aortic stenosis, valve area (cm^2)

Mild	>1.2
Moderate	0.5 – 1.2
Severe	<0.5

II. Aortic insufficiency, pressure half-times (m/s)

Mild	>500
Moderate	200 – 500
Severe	<200

III. Mitral stenosis, valve area (cm^2)

Mild	>1.8
Moderate	1.3 – 1.8
Severe	<1.3

IV. Mitral stenosis, pressure half-times (m/s)

Mild	<180
Moderate	180 – 280
Severe	>280

GLOSSARY

Aliasing — A phenomenon which occurs in a pulsed Doppler system when the frequency shift (or Doppler shift) exceeds the Nyquist limit (1/2 PRF) and is demonstrated on a spectral display by ambiguous velocities.

Angle of incidence — The angle (usually designated θ or theta) between the ultrasonic beam and the path of the moving target(s).

Bandwidth — The net difference between the highest and lowest frequencies on a given spectral tracing.

Bernoulli equation — The equation from which is derived the pressure difference between two points along a streamline.

Color Doppler — The superimposition of Color-coded imaging of blood flow on two-dimensional echocardiographic images.

Confined jet — A discrete area of flow which is distal to a constriction (or obstruction), composed of increased velocities (compared to upstream flow).

Continuity equation — The equation which is derived from the principle of conservation of mass. In a steady flow system, it describes the equality of flow between two points, despite changes in the velocity or area of this system.

Continuous wave (CW) Doppler — The simultaneous transmitting and receiving of ultrasonic waves using two transducers.

Doppler effect — A perceived change in the original frequency due to relative motion between the source and reflector.

Doppler shift — The net difference between the transmitted and received frequency.

Hertz (Hz) — Equivalent to cycles per second, both terms used to designate the units for frequency.

High PRF — Pulse repetition frequencies (see **PRF**) higher (2 to 4 times) than that which is used in standard pulsed Doppler, thus increasing maximum measurable velocities.

Laminar flow — A characteristic of flow through a circular tube or vessel which is parallel (or in the same radial position), free of turbulence, and producing a narrow bandwidth.

Modified Bernoulli equation — A simplified version of the Bernoulli equation which eliminates the acceleration and viscous terms and is applicable to most of the flow conditions in the heart and great vessels.

Multigate Doppler — The analysis of frequencies of multiple sample volumes along a single ultrasonic beam, utilized in flow imaging.

Nyquist limit — The maximum detectable frequency in a given pulsed Doppler system, equal to one half of the PRF.

Packet size — Another term for processing time.

Pressure half-time — The time that it takes for the pressure (in a steady flow system) to decrease or drop to one half of its initial value.

Pulse repetition frequency (PRF) — The rate of transmission of an ultrasonic beam.

Range — The distance (in cm) between the transducer and a specific point (or depth) that undergoes frequency analysis.

Range ambiguity — The inability of continuous-wave Doppler to localize a range (see **Range**) along the ultrasonic beam.

Range-gating — The use of a variable time delay to vary the range (see **Range**) along the ultrasonic beam of a transducer.

Sample volume — The region of flow (or volume) which undergoes frequency analysis in pulsed Doppler.

Turbulent (variant) flow — The characteristic of flow which is nonuniform in velocity and/or direction.

Velocity limit — The maximum measurable velocity (without aliasing) in a pulsed Doppler system. Also analagous to the Nyquist limit.

INDEX

U

V

W